OPTIMAL
DETOX

*How to Cleanse Your Body
of Colloidal and Crystalline Toxins*

CHRISTOPHER VASEY, N.D.

TRANSLATED BY JON E. GRAHAM

Healing Arts Press
Rochester, Vermont • Toronto, Canada

Healing Arts Press
One Park Street
Rochester, Vermont 05767
www.HealingArtsPress.com

SUSTAINABLE FORESTRY INITIATIVE Certified Sourcing
www.sfiprogram.org
SFI-00854

Text stock is SFI certified

Healing Arts Press is a division of Inner Traditions International

Originally published in French under the title *Détoxication optimale: Gérez et éliminez vos colles et cristaux* by Éditions Jouvence, www.editions-jouvence.com, info@editions-jouvence.com
First U.S. edition published in 2013 by Healing Arts Press

Note to the reader: *This book is intended as an informational guide. The remedies, approaches, and techniques described herein are meant to supplement, and not to be a substitute for, professional medical care or treatment. They should not be used to treat a serious ailment without prior consultation with a qualified health care professional.*

Library of Congress Cataloging-in-Publication Data

Vasey, Christopher.
  [Dètoxication optimale. English]
  Optimal detox : how to cleanse your body of colloidal and crystalline toxins / Christopher Vasey. — 1st U.S. ed.
    p. cm.
  Includes index.
  Summary: "A practical guide to identifying and targeting toxins with the most appropriate and effective detox methods"—Provided by publisher
  ISBN 978-1-59477-489-8 (pbk.) — ISBN 978-1-62055-143-1 (e-book)
  1. Detoxification (Health) I. Title.
  RA784.5.V3713 2013
  613.2—dc23

                                                        2012027366

Printed and bound in the United States by Lake Book Manufacturing, Inc. The text stock is SFI certified. The Sustainable Forestry Initiative® program promotes sustainable forest management.

10 9 8 7 6 5 4 3 2 1

Text design and layout by Brian Boynton
This book was typeset in Garamond Premier Pro with ITC Legacy Sans and Sabon as display fonts

Photo credits: page 4, Adam Gregor; page 8, Christopher Vasey; page 24, endostock; page 67, Lev Olkha; page 73, anna; page 107, margouillat; page 21, A-L-N-O-O-R; page 150, omicron; page 154, RG; page 35, Tomo Jesenicnik; page 1 and 164, Yuri Arcurs.

To send correspondence to the author of this book, mail a first-class letter to the author c/o Inner Traditions • Bear & Company, One Park Street, Rochester, VT 05767, and we will forward the communication, or visit the author's website at **www.christophervasey.ch/EN/HOME.html.**

OPTIMAL
DETOX

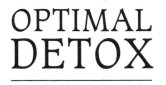

"Christopher Vasey has once again written an important book that advances our understanding of health and gives readers a clear approach to detoxification that far surpasses the majority of books in this realm. He offers the layperson masterful insights that are based on real-world clinical experience, traditional wisdom, and straightforward science. Dr. Vasey is a brilliant spokesperson for the naturopathic approach. This is a concise, readable, and practical book that puts the power to heal into your own hands. Highly recommended."

MARC DAVID, NUTRITIONAL PSYCHOLOGIST, FOUNDER OF
THE INSTITUTE FOR THE PSYCHOLOGY OF EATING, AND
AUTHOR OF *THE SLOW DOWN DIET* AND *NOURISHING WISDOM*

"Christopher Vasey, N.D., perfectly explains the major importance of a well-balanced biological terrain as well as the need to control the effects of external pollutants (free radicals, heavy metals, chemical additives in foods, chemical molecules in medicines, etc.) and internal pollutants: colloidal and crystalline wastes. These modern toxins do not have biologically programmed "exit routes." Our body, infinitely adaptable for millennia, has not had the necessary time to adapt to these toxic wastes. *Optimal Detox* offers the tools to live a healthier and more youthful life. I highly recommend this book."

YANN ROUGIER, M.D., AUTHOR OF *DELTA MEDICINE* AND
FOUNDING MEMBER OF THE INSTITUTE FOR APPLIED
NEURONUTRITION AND NEUROSCIENCES

Contents

Introduction   1

1   Toxins and Disease   4

2   Colloidal and Crystalline Toxins   24

3   The Different Eliminatory Organs for Colloidal and Crystalline Toxins   34

4   The Different Illnesses Caused by Colloidal and Crystalline Toxins   67

5   Food Sources of Colloidal and Crystalline Toxins   107

6   Drainage Methods   123

7   Regulating Your Food Intake   154

Conclusion   164

Index   166

Introduction

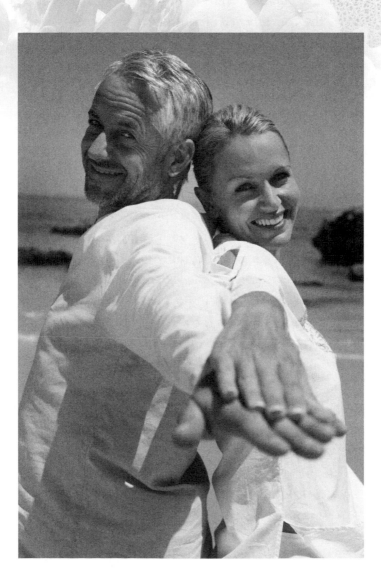

The times in which we live are characterized by many forms of chemical pollution and a tendency by many people to overeat, the consequence of which is that a wide variety of harmful substances are constantly entering our bodies. These substances, alone or in combination with others, are the basis for most illnesses.

From the natural medicine perspective it is the accumulation of toxins in the body that is the primary cause of health disorders. They thicken the blood, clog the blood vessels, and cause congestion in the organs, which creates inflammation and hardening that disrupts their proper functioning. It is logical then that the therapy and preventive health measures would concentrate on dealing with toxins: controlling their entry and encouraging their elimination.

Although extensive knowledge of these substances can be very useful in certain cases, in practice it is most often unnecessary. In fact, as varied as the different toxins may appear to be, they can all be divided into two major groups: the colloidal and crystalline toxins that are the subject of this book.

Each of these groups consists of toxins that share generally similar characteristics, are eliminated by the same excretory organs, and engender diseases that are similar in nature, which thus require fundamentally identical treatments.

This information, which is still not commonly known, can provide enormous assistance because it allows more effective treatment to be employed when choosing:

- Which eliminatory organs need to be stimulated first
- Which foods to monitor, as producers of one of these two kinds of toxins

The purpose of this book is to provide a comprehensive picture of these two major waste categories in order to optimize their drainage from the body, which in turn will encourage a return to good health.

1

Toxins and Disease

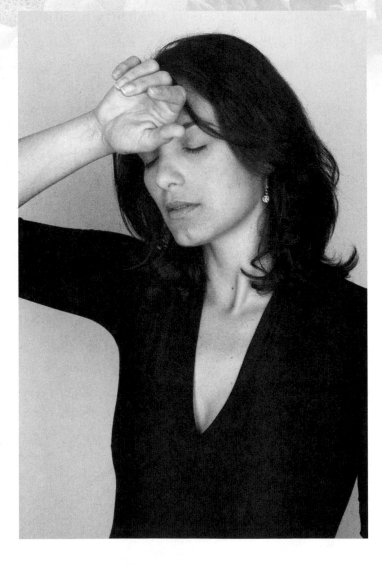

What are the true causes of diseases?

At first glance, one would think that the causes are as numerous and diverse as the diseases themselves. Doesn't every disease have its own characteristics, a different way of starting, developing, and evolving? The number of germs and poisons is immense as are the possibilities of hormonal, glandular, enzymatic, and immune system deficiencies.

However, careful observation will show that, fundamentally, all illnesses share one cause: the deterioration of the terrain, the body's internal cellular environment. This is not a new discovery. Hippocrates, the father of medicine, taught it thousands of years ago.

> Disease has one fundamental cause: the deterioration of the biological terrain.

THE TERRAIN

This word *terrain* has the same meaning as when we talk about the soil out of which a plant grows. The terrain is more or less fertile, acidic, compact, and so forth. It is thereby favorable or unfavorable to the growth of a particular plant. The same is true of the terrain in the human body. Of course, our organs do not consist of plants but of cells. Cells are the tiniest life units inside our bodies. Like all other living things, they must inhabit an environment with characteristics that are suitable for them. For cells, this environment is fluid rather than solid. First and foremost, we must understand that there are two different fluids with which they are in direct contact. The first is intracellular fluid, in other words the fluid that fills the insides of cells. It is home to the core and the organs of the cell (the organelles). Our bodies primarily consist of intracellular fluid as it represents 50 percent of our body weight.

The other fluid our cells are in direct contact with is that in which they are immersed: extracellular serum. This forms the immediate exterior environment of the cell. Quantitatively speaking, this fluid represents 15 percent of the weight of the body.

These two fluids, on which the cells are dependent for their nutrient supply and the elimination of their wastes, hence their very survival, form what we call the terrain. There are also two more fluids with which the cells have indirect contact: lymph and blood. The body weight of these two fluids together is 5 percent.

BODY FLUID LEVELS AND THEIR BODY WEIGHT PERCENTAGE

Fluid	Percent of Body Weight
Blood and Lymph	5%
Extracellular Fluid	15%
Intracellular Fluid	50%

Blood circulates through the blood vessels. These vessels branch off into finer and finer threads as they wend their way through the body, reducing in size to the diameter of a hair, from which their name of capillaries is derived (*capillaris* is the Latin word for hair). These capillaries make their way into the depths of the tissues. Although they never enter the cells, they do traverse their immediate vicinity, and they carry the blood charged with the oxygen and nutrients the cells require. Crossing through the extremely fine walls of the capillaries, the nutrients enter the extracellular fluid. It is here where the cells can absorb these nutrients. A movement in the opposite direction also occurs. The toxins rejected by the cells enter the extracellular fluid, from which they make their way into the capillaries. These vessels then carry the toxins to the eliminatory organs, such as the kidneys and liver.

The extracellular fluid is created from the blood. Blood is formed of fairly large solid elements—red corpuscles, for example—and a fluid part: blood serum. Leaving the blood corpuscles behind, the serum can cross through the capillary walls and reach the cell's outer environment. The composition of the blood serum is similar to that of the extracellular fluid. Its contribution allows the extracellular fluid to maintain its volume and to regenerate.

The second fluid in indirect contact with the cells is the lymph. This fluid is created from the extracellular fluid. Its composition is practically the same. Their similarities are so great that extracellular serum is often described as being lymph.

Lymph is a whitish fluid that circulates through the lymphatic vessels. These vessels start in the depths of the tissues as extremely thin threads. As they join together they form vessels of increasingly larger diameter. They traverse the lymphatic ganglions and eventually spill their lymph into the bloodstream at the level of the subclavian veins (at the base of the throat). Lymph therefore moves in a one-way direction: from the depths of the body to the surface. It carries the wastes expelled by the cells, as well as dead germs and worn-out parts of the cells, into the bloodstream. Once they have been added to the blood, these wastes are carried to the eliminatory organs to be expelled from the body.

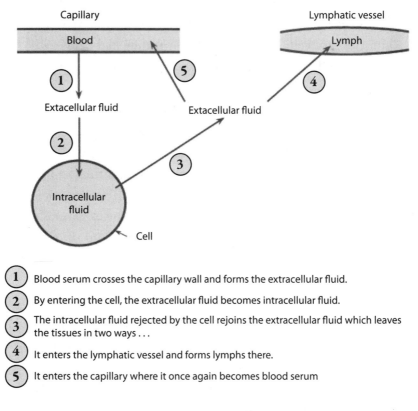

① Blood serum crosses the capillary wall and forms the extracellular fluid.

② By entering the cell, the extracellular fluid becomes intracellular fluid.

③ The intracellular fluid rejected by the cell rejoins the extracellular fluid which leaves the tissues in two ways . . .

④ It enters the lymphatic vessel and forms lymphs there.

⑤ It enters the capillary where it once again becomes blood serum

Fig 1.1. The circulation of bodily fluids

The cells are therefore immersed in an ocean consisting of different liquids and are entirely dependent on these fluids. In fact, cells do not enjoy the ability to move to the boundaries of the body to obtain their necessary oxygen and nutrients and to expel their wastes, which is essential if they are to keep their life center safe and healthy. The cells remain in their place, and it is these different fluids that bring the "outside" to the "inside."

> The intracellular and extracellular fluids, the blood, and the lymph form the terrain in which our bodies' cells can prosper or not, depending upon the characteristics of this terrain.

TERRAIN AND HEALTH

There is an ideal composition of the terrain viewed as a whole. It provides the cells and organs an optimal resistance capacity and vitality; health in other words. What results from this is that any deviation from this composition can compromise health, and the greater the change, the greater the opportunity for disease to develop and become serious.

The composition of the terrain can be altered in two different ways. The first is that certain substances (vitamins, minerals, and so forth) that should be found in the terrain are not there in sufficient quantity or are completely absent. In this case diseases of deficiencies appear. They can be treated by providing the body with the nutrients it lacks, which is above all the role of nutritherapy or nutrition.

The second possibility is that certain substances exist in excess of the ideal composition. These can either be substances that are normally found in the body, but not at such high levels (uric acid, urea), or substances that do not normally form part of the composition of the terrain (toxic food additives, medications, and poisons created by pollution).

In this second case, the diseases that are caused are the result of an excess.

It is this second cause, the overload of toxins as the starting point of illness, that is the main focus of this book. The subject of deficiencies will not be discussed further as we are going to concentrate solely on toxins from this point forward.

☞ Good to Know

The word *overload* is not used as it would be in the case of excess weight, or overweight. Instead it refers to the overload of wastes, toxins, and poisons in the terrain. This can exist even in cases where excess weight is not an issue.

THE TWO CAUSES OF TERRAIN DETERIORATION

Overload of Toxins	Excess of uric acid, urea, cholesterol, acids
Nutrient Deficiencies	Lack of nutrients such as vitamins, minerals, trace elements, and amino acids

TOXINS AND DISEASE

How do toxins make us sick? The idea that toxins could play a role in causing disease might appear to be surprising, but if you think about it, it is perfectly logical. The human body is primarily made up of liquid. Fluids represent 70 percent of our body weight. These fluids circulate throughout all our tissues. An overly large presence of toxins will cause them to become less fluidic, which in turn slows down their circulation. The result of this is a deficiency in the transport of nutrients, hormones, and lymphocytes on the one hand, and the transport of toxins on the other.

When they are numerous, toxins produce effects that are harmful to our health. They thicken the blood, clog and block the blood vessels, cause congestion in the organs, cause blockages in the joints, create sedimentation (kidney and gall stones), and waterproof the mucous membranes, preventing their proper function. The disruptions caused by this toxic oversaturation account for one aspect of health disorders. Another aspect comes from the defensive reactions triggered by the body to rid itself of these toxins. The body does not remain a passive bystander when it is invaded by a mass of wastes. Instead it reacts by looking for ways to eliminate as many of these as possible, as quickly as it can. The effects of this can be seen on the skin in the form of pimples and eczema; in the lungs by colds, sinusitis, and bronchitis; in the digestive tract by episodes of diarrhea, hemorrhoids, gallbladder flushes, and so forth. The illnesses listed above, which are generally considered to be diseases in and of themselves, are therefore really symptoms of cleansing crises or detoxifications that the body initiates intentionally, and which are sometimes joined by a microbial infection.

> The body does not remain a passive bystander when
> it is invaded by a mass of wastes.

Toxins can also have negative effects that are not caused by their quantity but by the aggressive nature of their substance. Some wastes have, in fact, a corrosive or irritating effect on the mucous membranes of the organs and cells. They injure and inflame them, which in turn causes other kinds of health disorders.

It is not only logical that toxins are a basic cause of disease; *it is also a fact that can be easily observed as in the following instances.*

- Phlegm is eliminated from the body when a person is suffering from asthma, bronchitis, laryngitis, coughs, sinusitis, and the common cold.
- Wastes overload the glands of the skin and flow outward in the form of all sorts of pimples and eczema.
- Fat residues thicken the blood, become deposited on the vessel walls (arteriosclerosis), or block the blood vessels (heart attacks and strokes).
- Joints become painful and make a grinding sound because of the grit that has collected there.
- Undesirable substances are ejected from the upper end of the digestive tract (vomiting) or the lower end (diarrhea).
- Wastes appear in excess amounts in the urine and irritate the urinary tract (burning sensation), form sediment (urinary stones), or cause lesions that harm

the mucous membranes, which allow germs to get settled there and trigger infections.

• Among the undesirable substances that can make us sick, we should also include uric acid (gout), salt (edema, high blood pressure), excessive sugar (diabetes), and carcinogens, which can form tumors, and so forth.

Toxins that disturb and harm the body, and which it tries to expel, can be found in every disease.

WHERE DO TOXINS COME FROM?

The origin of toxins can be found first and foremost in the individual's diet. When the body receives more nutrients than it needs, some of them will remain unused. They overburden the terrain to no purpose, and although they have nutritious value, they can therefore be considered as toxins. Furthermore, overeating will exhaust the digestive tract. Over time, digestion will become worse and worse. The foods eaten are not broken down for their nutrients but instead ferment and rot. The result will be more wastes overloading the terrain. Added to these wastes will be those that result from the normal use of proteins, fats, and carbohydrates. In fact, the normal breakdown of proteins will produce wastes like urea and uric acid. The breaking down of fats will create saturated fatty acids, cholesterol, and so forth.

Diet is the primary cause of toxins.

The task of the body's eliminatory organs, such as the kidneys and liver, is to rid the body of these toxins. They do this by filtering them out of the bloodstream and expelling them out of the body in the form of stools, urine, and sweat. But this cleansing process will only be performed correctly if the eliminatory organs are able to follow the same body rhythm that produces the wastes. *When we overeat, the wastes that the body produces are greater than the capacity of the body to eliminate them.* The consequence of this is that some of these wastes are not eliminated and remain in the body, thereby causing a deterioration of the terrain.

FACTORS THAT CONTRIBUTE TO FOULING OF THE TERRAIN

- Overeating
- Intestinal fermentation
- Nutrient utilization
- Insufficient eliminations

In addition to the wastes that come from the foods we eat and can be considered legitimate, there are a host of other wastes that should not be in our bodies. They have no nutritional value, and the body does not have a cycle in place for their removal. This group of wastes includes insecticides, herbicides, fungicides, and other chemicals used to treat agricultural products. A portion of these substances becomes imbedded in the tissues of the foods we eat. Food additives, such as colorings, thickening agents, preservatives, and antioxidants, which are even poisonous in part, can also be added to this category. Altogether they create a chemical fouling of the terrain. Other harmful substances can enter the terrain and damage it during the consumption of stimulants (coffee, tea, tobacco), alcohol, drugs, and medications. The pollution of our air, water, and soil is another source of the poisons that have combined with those already mentioned.

ORIGIN OF TOXINS

- Food
- Products for treating food such as herbicides and pesticides
- Food additives such as coloring agents and preservatives
- Stimulants such as coffee, tea, and tobacco
- Medications and drugs
- Pollution

HOW ARE WASTES ELIMINATED?

The normal functioning of the body inevitably produces wastes. Our bodies are therefore naturally equipped with the means of eliminating these wastes. Five organs, known as the eliminatory or excretory organs, together with the female sexual organs are intended to filter these wastes out of the bloodstream and expel them from the body.

These organs are:

- The liver. It expels the wastes diluted in the bile. This latter substance is simultaneously a digestive juice and a support substance for the elimination of toxins.
- The intestines. By means of stools, they evacuate the substances the body has not assimilated (bran and thick vegetable fiber) as well as the toxins that enter the bowels through the intestinal walls.

- The kidneys. They evacuate the toxins contained in the urine.
- The skin. The sudoriferous and sebaceous glands secrete sweat and sebum, respectively, two support substances for the elimination of toxins.
- The lungs. An organ that specializes in the elimination of gaseous wastes (carbon dioxide) but that also provides relief to the other eliminatory organs by evacuating fluid wastes in the form of phlegm.

The eliminatory organs are only overtaxed when we eat too much and thereby produce more toxins than these organs can normally expel from the body.

🖐 Good to Know

There are two kinds of detox: one is the elimination of the toxins naturally produced by the body such as uric acid, urea, and so forth. The other refers to the elimination of toxic substances (heavy metals, plant-based poisons, drugs, medications).

THERAPY

In natural medicine the purpose of the therapy is to remove the cause of the disease. More on this therapeutic path can be found in my book *The Naturopathic Way*. Given that, from the naturopathic perspective, illness is the result of an accumulation of wastes and toxins in the terrain, there are two essential steps that must be taken.

- Halt the arrival of new toxins.
- Eliminate toxins that are already in the terrain.

The situation can be compared to what happens when a bathtub has been filled with too much water; it will overflow and flood the house. How are we to prevent this? There are two things we must do. One of them consists of removing the plug from the drain so that the water can flow out of the tub. However, there is a risk that this step will not be enough, because the outflow of water down the drain is less than the amount that continues to come in through the tap. Thus a second measure proves necessary: turn off the faucet. These two measures taken together will allow us to avoid disaster. The same is true when speaking of the human body. Not only must we get rid of the toxins that have already collected in the terrain but also take steps to prevent the influx of new toxins that continue to saturate and damage it. Let's go over these two points in greater detail.

Shut Off the Source of the Toxins

The principal source of toxins is our diet. *If an illness has appeared, it is because the foods we consume supply and produce a greater quantity of toxins than our eliminatory organs can remove.* It is therefore imperative to reduce our consumption. This can be a broad restriction. The main goal is to reduce the intake of all foodstuffs. In this way we counter general overeating with a generalized restriction. But the restriction can also target much more specific food categories. For example, one may seek to generally reduce the consumption of fats, meats, or sugars. This involves specific restrictions that are implemented to counter the overconsumption of clearly defined foodstuffs. The rest of the individual's diet may be perfectly normal and healthy, and it is the overeating of one single kind of food that is responsible for the fouling of the terrain.

The degree of restriction can vary. It can be light when the clogged state of the terrain is not very pronounced. Conversely, the dietary restriction can be quite severe, involving even total abstinence from a particular food, when a massive overload exists and the resulting health problems require urgent attention.

The Elimination of Those Toxins Already Present

To restore health, the terrain that has been overloaded with toxins must be cleared of the wastes that have collected there. The only path that these toxins can use to leave the body is that provided by the eliminatory organs: the liver, kidneys, intestines, skin, and respiratory tract. These are in fact the only organs in our bodies that have the ability to cleanse the blood of wastes and to carry them out of the body.

> The only path that toxins can use to leave the body
> is that provided by the eliminatory organs.

When the terrain is overloaded, the eliminatory organs are generally fatigued and cannot function at full capacity. They must therefore be stimulated and sustained so they may recover their normal working rhythm. But simply implementing this measure is not enough. It only allows the elimination process to return to normal, but it does not help it catch up with what collected when the organs were not working normally. To achieve this second goal—catching up with the excess accumulation of wastes—it is essential to make the eliminatory organs work at a higher rate than normal. By doing this, over time, not only will the daily accumulation of toxins be eliminated, but so will those that collected in the past.

The stimulation of the eliminatory organs can be achieved by:

- Taking medicinal plants (hepatic or diuretic herbs)
- Hydrotherapy (warm baths, saunas)
- Massage of the appropriate reflex zones
- Physical exercise

ELIMINATING TOXINS FOR HEALING PURPOSES

Getting rid of toxins in order to preserve or restore health is a universal process. In the plant kingdom, for example, trees collect their metabolic wastes in their leaves. These toxin-charged leaves fall off in autumn when trees traditionally lose their leaves. This also takes place with conifers and indoor plants that regularly lose some of their thorns or leaves over the course of the year.

It is common knowledge that dogs and cats will eat grass to heal themselves of sickness. This is not just any kind of grass but particular kinds of herbs or grasses that have laxative, diuretic, or emetic properties. Apes and elephants do the same thing, but with different plants and sometimes with clay.

The blood purification cure performed with the help of purgative plants that folk healers recommend as an annual spring health procedure is along these same lines. This cure allows the body to get rid of the wastes produced by the richer and more concentrated foods we normally eat in winter. All the major religions have also advocated periods of diet or fasting as a means of forcing the body to burn away the toxins that have collected in its tissues. Sessions of intense sweating are practiced throughout the world for this purpose as well. We have the sauna in Nordic countries, the Arabic *hamman,* and the sweat lodge of Native Americans.

But, in addition to these folk practices, the greatest doctors throughout history have stated that the excess of toxins in the terrain constitutes the profound nature of disease. Hippocrates, the father of modern medicine, who lived two centuries before Christ, wrote: "All diseases are resolved either by the mouth, the bowels, the bladder, or some other such organ. Sweat is a common form of resolution in all these cases."

The seventeenth-century British doctor, Thomas Sydenham, who was nicknamed the English Hippocrates, stated: "A disease, however much its cause may be adverse to the human body, is nothing more than an effort of Nature, who strives with might and main to restore the health of the patient by the elimination of the morbific [disease-causing] humor."

Doctor Paul Carton, the pioneer of natural medicine in France at the beginning of the twentieth century, was equally convinced that "disease was the expression of an effort of purification."

Closer to the present day, Doctor Jean Seignalet wrote in his book *L'alimentation ou la troisième médicine* (Diet or the third medicine): "The extremely numerous food and bacterial molecules in the small intestine are, in my opinion, the primary culprits for 90 percent of diseases . . . barely curable if at all by standard methods."

Doctor Catherine Kousmine, meanwhile, also stated: "Whether it is cancer, chronic evolving polyarthritis, or multiple sclerosis, my basis treatment is the same. It involves eliminating as quickly as possible what I consider to be the source of disease, in other words poisoning . . . of intestinal origin."

THE TWO MAJOR KINDS OF TOXINS

A multitude of toxins, consequently, play an underlying role, either alone or in combination with others, in the creation of illness.

At first glance, we would think it necessary to be acquainted with every existing toxin as well as every illness it engenders in order to be able to take effective therapeutic action against it.

In practice, though, this knowledge is not essential. All toxins can, in fact, be divided into two major groups: the wastes called colloidal substances and those called crystals. Both groups include toxins that share many points in common. Their general characteristics are identical, the eliminatory organs that remove them are the same, and the diseases they cause are similar, as are the therapies they require for effective treatment.

📖 A Little History

The division of toxins into colloidal substances and crystals is due to the French naturopath Pierre-Valentin Marchesseau (1911–1994). He was one of the great pioneers and propagators of naturopathy in France and was possessed of a brilliant gift for synthesis. In 1940 he began to classify the confusing number of healing techniques into ten groups according to the natural agent upon which they were based. These are techniques involving food (dietetics, nutrition), water (hydrotherapy), air, movement, ideas (psychology), fluids (magnetism), rays (solar, color), reflexes, hands (massage), and plants (herbalism, aromatherapy). The treatments are structured into three cures: the detoxification cure, for ridding the body of the toxins that burden it; the revitalization cure, which regenerates the body by filling nutritional deficiencies; and the stabilization cure.

Pierre-Valentin Marchesseau wrote more than eighty booklets that present in a very helpful, synthesized way the various illnesses and the ways to treat them (www.spirvie-natura.fr). The official site for this great naturopath is www.marchesseau.fr.

A much greater therapeutic effectiveness can be obtained as a result of this classification, which is not well known even today, because it aids in choosing:

• Which eliminatory organs are to be stimulated as a matter of priority

- Which foods it is most important to monitor as producers of one of these two kinds of toxins

CONCLUSION

The natural medicine viewpoint is that illness is due primarily to an accumulation of toxins in the physiological terrain—the body's internal cellular environment. Thus the corresponding therapy consists of ridding the body of the wastes and poisons that attack it and hinder or disrupt its proper functioning.

2
Colloidal and Crystalline Toxins

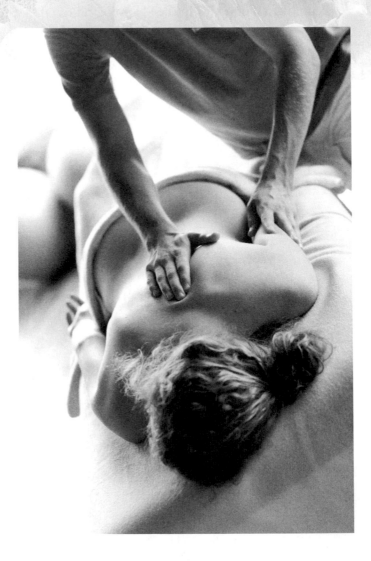

The terms *colloidal* and *crystalline* have been adopted because of their connection with a substance's ability or inability to cross through a semipermeable membrane. These membranes can be found throughout the body: on the cellular level, among the capillaries, and in the digestive and respiratory mucous membranes.

A membrane is a thin layer of cells. When they are permeable or semipermeable, their surface is pierced by a large number of small canals or pores that allow certain substances to pass from one side of the wall to the other. Whether a substance can pass through depends on the diameter of the substances dissolved in the fluids that are in contact with the membrane. There are two kinds of substances: those whose diameter is smaller than that of the canals, which ensures their easy passage, and those whose diameter is larger, which means they get held back.

Size is not the sole criterion that distinguishes between these two kinds of substances. As a general rule, those of small dimensions crystallize when the solution in which they have dissolved evaporates, hence their definition as crystalline substances. This is the case with sugar dissolved in water; syrup, for example. When it dries, syrup displays tiny sugar crystals. Similarly, when seawater is trapped in a small depression on a rock it will form salt crystals when the sun evaporates the liquid. Other substances, those that do not crystallize during evaporation, are of larger size. In the solid state, after their host solution has evaporated, they have a soft and amorphous appearance. These are known as colloidal substances because they are slimy and sticky. Examples of these substances are the gelatin dissolved in water or agar-agar in a fruit jelly.

What we have just said about these substances in general can be repeated concerning the toxins in the body. Some are of very small size and easily travel through the tissue membranes; these are crystals. The others are larger in size and have a hard time crossing through the body's filters. These are colloidal substances.

COLLOIDAL SUBSTANCES

Colloidal substances do not have a definite, consistent form. They are soft, malleable, and round; lacking any fixed structure. While their elastic consistency does not irritate the tissues, they hinder the organism and cause dysfunction because of their massive presence. They thicken their holding fluids, which include blood or lymph. This results in circulation slowing down and can even lead to clogged vessels. Colloidal toxins encumber the respiratory tract, more specifically the bronchia, the bronchioles, and the alveoli. They cause congestion in the organs and trigger a state of stasis, thereby obstructing the proper functioning of the organ.

It is easy for anyone to see if colloidal substances are present. Simply by blowing your nose in a handkerchief, you can see the viscous material that is expelled from your body. Another common source is spit or phlegm, the mucous substances that are coughed or expectorated from the body. The white-headed pimples of classic acne also secrete colloidal wastes. Pus, that often greenish or yellowish liquid produced by infections and inflammations (boils, earaches, cuts), is also a colloidal substance. Sometimes stools contain gray or brown mucus with a texture close to that of egg whites, capable of being stretched out. These, too, are colloidal wastes. The whitish layer that coats the tongue when we have a so-called furred tongue also consists of colloidal substances, just like the white discharges women release. Atheromas, which cannot be seen directly, but which are often mentioned with regard to cardiovascular diseases, are yellowish, lumpy fat deposits. They form on the interior walls of the blood vessels and, because of their characteristics, are also considered to be a form of colloidal waste. One of the most prominent characteristics of these substances is their lack of any fixed form.

> Colloidal substances do not irritate or assault the tissues but disrupt the organism and hinder its functioning.

Colloidal Substances from Fats

These are the most well known of the colloidal toxins, and their levels in the blood are frequently monitored.

- Cholesterol: This substance is produced by the body but is also carried into the organism by certain foods (eggs, butter, delicatessen meats). Cholesterol is beneficial when it is in the cells, where it can be utilized. Because it travels from one part of the body to another through the blood, it is normal for there to be a certain amount of cholesterol contained in the blood. But too high a level poses the risk of forming cholesterol deposits on the vessel walls and is harmful. The body no longer considers this cholesterol as a helpful substance but as a toxin of the colloidal group.

• Triglycerides: Like cholesterol, saturated fatty acids are useful to the body, but when overly concentrated they become harmful. They thicken the blood and form deposits (arteriosclerosis).

Colloidal Substances from Carbohydrates

These colloidal substances are not given specific names because their shape and composition is highly variable making them difficult to get a handle on. Although they are much less well known, their effects are just as harmful as those that originate from fats. The primary members of this family of colloidal wastes include:

• The flocculates—flakes of dead cells, dead germs, and toxins—blended into the protective mucus secreted by the mucous membranes, such as those of the respiratory system, for example.

• The collections of toxins, dead germs, and sebum secreted by the sebaceous glands.

• The residue of starches that have been insufficiently broken down. The starches that can be found in grains, breads, pasta, and so forth are made up of long chains of glucose molecules (sometimes as many as ten thousand molecules). Normally these chains are broken down into shorter and shorter chains during the digestive process until the smallest chains are broken down to their basic units: single glucose molecules. This process allows the body to use the energy provided by starch to the best advantage. But sometimes this dividing process does not work properly, leaving intact chains that can consist of thousands of molecules.

These then form viscous, shapeless heaps of colloidal substances, which will clog and foul the organism.

As noted above, colloidal toxins are not aggressive to the body, but they do disrupt its performance. A very common example of this disruption is the thickened blood in which colloidal wastes of fat and carbohydrate origin can be found. It is carrying more solid bodies than it should. This condition is extremely widespread today. To fight against the increase of blood viscosity and the risk of thrombosis—the forming of a blood clot in the veins—with the health problems that accompany it, medications called blood thinners are prescribed. The name of the remedy provides an accurate illustration of the situation: the blood is too dense and thick. This is caused by the presence of wastes, in this case colloidal toxins. To counter this, it is necessary to render the blood more liquid, more fluid.

CRYSTALS

The atoms that form crystals have the tendency to create definite geometric shapes as opposed to the amorphous, unstructured form of colloidal substances. These geometric shapes have the same straight lines and flat surfaces typical of rock crystals, sugar crystals, and salt crystals. This structure gives crystals their firmness and resistant qualities. They are rigid and capable of retaining their form under pressure.

Crystal wastes are smaller in size than a rock crystal, but the structure they share is the same. They are just as hard and have sharp edges, capable of cutting. This gives them an aggressive and irritating nature, hence their tendency to hurt the tissues and cause inflammations. Prolonged contact can even wound the host tissues—a wound known as a lesion.

During prolonged contact, crystals will cluster together. They then create crystalline structures that are larger in size, which are called stones, such as those that can be found in the kidneys or gallbladder.

Anyone can see the presence of crystalline wastes in the body. The sand particles we find in our eyes upon waking—and which are brought by the sandman according to legend—are crystals. It is also sand that we hear grinding in our joints, such as the sound we hear coming from the vertebra of the neck when we turn our head from left to right or right to left. When perspiration is highly concentrated, it will leave a dirty, powdery residue when it dries. These deposits are very tiny crystals. In comparison, the crystals that accumulate in the joints form deposits called tophi (the plural for tophus) that deform, obstruct, and inflame the joints. These tophi are responsible for illnesses such as gout. These are not the only examples of crystals to be found in the body. As we shall see in chapter 4, there are many others. The ones mentioned above, however, are among the easiest to observe.

The broad term *crystals* covers a specific, well-defined kind of waste product, whose names are certainly familiar to the reader. Most of them appear in the form of acids and are a by-product of the body's utilization of proteins. Crystals can also come from carbohydrates and fats, though.

Crystals are characterized by a structured, inflexible shape. They have an aggressive, irritating nature.

Crystalline Toxins from Proteins

- Uric acid: Purines, a protein substance contained in our cells and some foods (meat, coffee, soy), are transformed into uric acid so they can be expelled from the body.
- Urea: This toxin is the by-product of the breaking down of the amino acids in the cores of the cells.
- Creatinine: This is a by-product of the proteins connected with the wear and tear of the muscles.
- Oxalic acid: This acid can be found in a variety of vegetables, such as spinach, sorrel, and rhubarb, but the body also produces it in the utilization of certain amino acids.

Crystalline Toxins from Fats

- Acetoacetic acid (also called diacetic acid): This acid results from the improper metabolizing of fats and certain amino acids.
- Beta-hydroxybutyric acid: This is a waste product created when fats are not completely broken down.

Crystalline Toxins from Carbohydrates

- Pyruvic acid: This toxin results from the use and breakdown of glucose, especially from white sugar and white flour.
- Lactic acid: Glucose is burned during physical exercise and transformed into lactic acid.

Depleted Minerals

Minerals also play a role in the composition of tissues and secretions. After being used by the body, over time they will lose their electrical charge, in other words their vitality. At this point the body needs to eliminate them. Because of their crystalline structure, all minerals used up by the body are considered crystal wastes, but the primary emphasis falls upon those that are acids, including:

- Phosphorus
- Sulfur
- Chlorine

The public is familiar with the names of many specific crystal wastes, because their levels are among the things looked for in the analysis of blood or urine. Their presence in excess is considered to be the cause of disease.

TOXIN CHARACTERISTICS

	Colloidal	Crystalline
Size	Large	Small
Appearance	Rounded	Angular
Shape	Unstructured	Structured with corners and flat surfaces
Consistency	Soft	Hard
Harmful Effects	Congestion, obstruction	Inflammation, lesions
Physiological Example	Expelled phlegm	Grit that makes grinding noise in joints

	Colloidal	Crystalline
Chemical Example	Cholesterol	Uric acid
	Saturated fatty acids	Urea
	Starch residues	Creatinine
	Floculates	Various acids
		Used up minerals

CONCLUSION

There are two major categories of wastes: the colloidal toxins that are soft in consistency—such as phlegm—which cause congestion and blockages, and crystals that are hard in consistency and cause inflammation and even lesions in the tissues.

3

The Different Eliminatory Organs for Colloidal and Crystalline Toxins

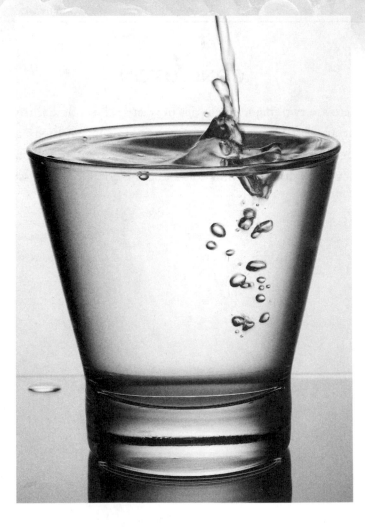

The removal of colloidal and crystalline wastes cannot be accomplished with equal effectiveness by just any eliminatory organ. Colloidal wastes have their own distinctive characteristics that are different from those of crystals. Consequently, these two kinds of wastes are filtered and eliminated by different organs.

The questions we now need to ask are: Which organs eliminate colloidal wastes? Which organs eliminate crystal wastes? and Why the distinction?

A WASTE PRODUCT'S SOLUBILITY OR INSOLUBILITY

The criteria that makes it possible to separate these two categories of toxins, and thereby determine which organs will remove them, is whether they are soluble in a liquid.

Crystals are water soluble. Therefore they can dissolve in various bodily fluids such as blood, serum, and urine. Although they possess a firm consistency, crystals will easily dissolve in water where they lose their solidity and rigidity. They make the transition from a solid state to a fluid one just like the salt or sugar that is blended with a liquid. Before they are immersed in water, grains of salt are visible and still possess their crystalline structure. Once they have been mixed with water, they not only become invisible but lose the hardness that made it possible to feel them. This ability to dissolve makes it possible for them to easily travel through the filter of the eliminatory organs. This is also helped by the fact that crystal wastes are naturally small in size.

Colloidal substances, on the other hand, start off much larger than crystals. Furthermore, they are not soluble in liquids. While they will become somewhat diluted on contact with water, they do not dissolve. They retain their soft consistency and thus remain both visible and palpable. This can easily be observed by spitting or sneezing into water. These mucous substances, which are colloidal toxins, do not separate into smaller and smaller particles that eventually melt and disappear in the liquid. Instead, they remain in the form of visible, tangible masses. Because of their size, these masses cannot easily pass through the filters of the eliminatory organs and they tend to be retained by these filters.

ELIMINATION WITH OR WITHOUT LIQUID

The characteristics of crystals ensure that they are easily transported by water. They are therefore eliminated by those organs that use a liquid support medium in order to evacuate wastes from the body: the kidneys and the sudoriferous glands that, with urine and perspiration, respectively, provide an abundant amount of fluid for transporting crystals.

THE ELIMINATION OF CRYSTALS
(WITH A LIQUID SUPPORT MEDIUM)

Eliminatory Organs	Secretions
Kidneys	Urine
Sudoriferous glands	Perspiration

Colloidal wastes, meanwhile, are not water soluble. They will therefore be eliminated from the body by those organs that use a support medium that is not so fluid, in other words one that is more viscous in nature to which these substances can bind. These organs are:

- The liver, which secretes bile, a thick digestive juice that is viscous and runny in appearance
- The intestines, which evacuate the relatively solid materials that make up stools
- The sebaceous glands, which secrete sebum, a thick, oily coating intended to lubricate the skin
- The respiratory tract, which primarily evacuates wastes in a gaseous form but can also provide an emergency exit for more solid forms of waste such as phlegm and expectorations (the mucous substances that can be coughed or spit out of the body)
- Vaginal mucous membranes, which serve as another emergency exit for eliminating wastes in the form of white discharges

THE ELIMINATION OF COLLOIDAL TOXINS
(WITHOUT A LIQUID SUPPORT MEDIUM)

Eliminatory Organs	Secretions
Liver	Bile
Intestines	Stools
Sebaceous glands	Sebum
Respiratory tract	Phlegm, mucus
Vaginal mucous membranes	White discharges

We will now take a detailed look at how these two different eliminatory organ groups extract and filter waste from the bloodstream. We shall also examine how they eliminate these wastes.

We will examine the eliminatory organs in the order outlined in the following table.

TOXINS AND THEIR ELIMINATORY ORGANS

Toxin	Eliminatory Organ
Colloidal wastes	Liver
	Intestines
	Sebaceous glands
	Lungs
Crystals	Kidneys
	Sudoriferous glands

THE ELIMINATORY ORGANS FOR COLLOIDAL WASTES

The Liver

The liver is one of the largest organs in the body. It measures on average 28 centimeters (around 11 inches) going from left to right, 16 centimeters (6¼ inches) thick, and 8 centimeters (just over 3⅛ inches) high. It is located in the rib cage beneath the right lung. Because it is protected by the ribs, only a very small portion of it can be touched. The liver has very high cellular density. Its weight in a dead body is 1.5 kilograms (a little more than 3 pounds) but when still full of blood in a living individual, its weight is closer to 2.5

kilograms (around 5½ pounds). More than a liter and a half of blood passes through the liver every minute; a significant amount, exemplifying the importance of this organ.

The liver is distinguished from the other organs of the body by the multiple duties it performs. It plays an active role in the regulation of glycemia, the mineral and protein levels in the bloodstream, and so forth. It is also active in the synthesis of proteins and fats, and bile formation, among other tasks. But the functions it performs that concern us here are those related to its ability to eliminate toxins.

The functions of the liver related to the elimination of toxins are as follows:

- Purifies the bloodstream of wastes and cellular metabolic residues: fats and poorly broken-down starches, surplus cholesterol, dead cells, and depleted minerals
- Neutralizes the poisons created by intestinal fermentation and putrefaction
- Kills germs and viruses, and neutralizes the toxins they produce
- Neutralizes and deactivates many toxic substances: food additives, chemically synthesized products used in gardening (herbicides, pesticides), medications, heavy metals, poisons, by-products of pollution

All of these wastes are expelled by the liver along with the substances it produces to digest the fats. Bile is therefore both a digestive juice and a support medium for the elimination of toxins. These latter substances are mixed with the bolus (the food mass ingested by the body after it has been chewed) to be evacuated with the stools.

> Bile is both a digestive juice and a support medium
> for the elimination of toxins.

The toxins filtered by the liver are brought there by the bloodstream. One source of this blood is the aorta; this blood is the oxygen-rich blood the heart gets from the lungs. It is nonetheless charged with the toxins that the cells have rejected. The other primary source of this blood is the portal vein, which carries the blood flowing from the intestines. This blood is loaded with fats and carbohydrates, as well as the poisons introduced into the body by food (additives, pollution) or those that are created by intestinal fermentation. After entering the liver, both the aorta vein and the portal vein branch off into many smaller vessels resembling the branches of a tree. These vessels become tinier and tinier and make close contact with the hepatic cells. Eventually they empty their contents in the microscopic spaces that are located between the rows of cells. These spaces, which are called sinusoidal spaces, are where the blood purification takes place. Wastes are extracted from the bloodstream not through a simple passive filtering but through an active process of capturing, neutralizing, transforming, and then concentrating them before excreting them in the form of bile.

The wastes filtered by the hepatic cells are released into minuscule conduits called bile capillaries, or canaliculi. These canaliculi join together to form larger channels, the right and left hepatic ducts. These ducts then merge together to form a single channel, the common hepatic duct. This channel carries bile into the digestive tract. The gallbladder is adjacent to this duct. It serves as a reservoir in which some of the bile produced by the liver is stored during digestive intervals.

The accumulated bile permits the body to maintain sufficient amounts of this substance to digest fats, even when they arrive in great quantity, as is the case during a meal. In order to increase its effectiveness, bile is concentrated during its stay in the gallbladder. When enough bile has concentrated in the gallbladder, bile coming from the liver goes directly into the choledochal duct, the name given to the hepatic duct from the junction that connects it to the gallbladder.

The liver can produce anywhere from 1 to 1.5 liters of bile daily. While it is still in the liver, bile is about 97 percent water. After concentration in the gallbladder, this amount goes down to 84 percent. It is therefore a viscous liquid. Its thickness makes it runny, meaning that individual drops do not separate when it flows but remain stuck together as if on a thread. Its characteristics resemble those of colloidal wastes, and the liver is, in fact, one of the eliminatory

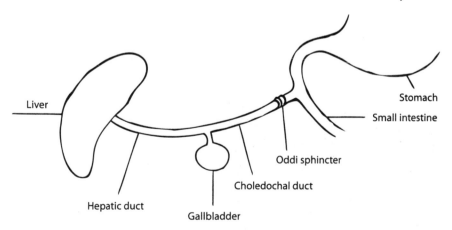

Fig. 3.1. The liver and the bile ducts

organs for removing colloidal toxins from the body. Bile has a very bitter taste, and its color ranges from golden yellow to a brownish green. It is largely made up of substances originating from fats and can easily transport the aggregates of improperly broken-down starches.

The work the liver does purifying the bloodstream largely depends on how well that blood is circulating. The normal blood flow through the liver is about 1.5 liters per minute. This flow can be reduced, however. This occurs with individuals who are sedentary and do not perform much physical activity, or when the production of wastes becomes too excessive as happens with individuals who overeat. The bloodstream thickens and becomes sluggish, creating poor circulation so the liver receives less oxygen. It is consequently less capable of working properly while the toxin-laden blood it is receiving demands even more effective action than usual. Two harmful situations are the result. The first is that the liver begins collecting in its tissues some of the wastes it is receiving instead of eliminating them. When this occurs we describe the liver as congested. The filter has been clogged or greatly obstructed. Second, the unpurified blood flows back into general circulation by side paths. Instead of being expelled from the body, the wastes carried by this blood are placed back in the tissues where they become deposited in the cellular fluids and lymph and contribute to the overall deterioration of the terrain.

A congested liver is one whose tissues have collected some of the wastes it has received but has not been able to eliminate.

Poor elimination of waste can also occur due to weakness in the bile ducts. The process of expelling bile out of the gallbladder is a very active one. The muscles in the wall of this organ strongly contract and force the bile out of its pocket. However, the gallbladder cannot eject bile very easily if it is too thick. This is the case when it is overladen with wastes, mainly colloidal wastes. Furthermore, when people overeat, the large, thick bile mass they produce will stretch the walls of the gallbladder. Over time, these walls begin to sag (gallbladder ptosis). The muscles of the wall lose their tone and are no longer capable of contracting strongly enough to force the bile out of the gallbladder.

Thick bile has an additional inconvenience. The wastes it contains begin to collect into small masses. While they are still small, they are described as *grit* or *sand*. But when these individual gritty masses combine together, they form gallstones. These lumps of concentrated colloidal toxins can become as large as walnuts and equally as hard. This compromises the ability of bile to flow through the bile ducts and thereby makes the elimination of toxins more difficult. Bile stagnation in the liver and gallbladder permits bilirubin, the pigment that gives bile its yellow color, to enter the bloodstream. It then travels throughout the body causing the skin and the whites of the eyes to take on a slight yellowish coloration in individuals with weakened livers. This coloration becomes much more intense in individuals suffering from hepatitis.

Stagnation of the bile in the gallbladder and bile ducts is not only due to overeating and a sedentary lifestyle. Nervous tension, anxiety, and stress can also bring about this condition. The exit of the choledochal duct, which carries bile into the intestine, is controlled by a muscular valve, the Oddi sphincter (also known as the sphincter of ampulla). This muscle surrounds the entire exit orifice of this duct. By contracting or relaxing, it ensures that this duct opens and closes in accordance with the body's requirements. This muscle is governed by a nerve, and if an individual is under a lot of nervous stress the information flow to the muscle will be disrupted causing it to spasm. If the entrance that allows bile to enter the intestines remains closed too often this causes the bile—as well as the wastes it contains—to remain trapped in the bile ducts, where it stagnates. These types of inadequate liver function are known as hepatic insufficiency.

CAUSES OF HEPATIC INSUFFICIENCY
- Overeating
- Sedentary lifestyle
- Poor blood circulation
- Nervous tension
- Stress

It should be noted that when the liver has been over-worked for too long a period, it will have greater and greater difficulty performing its duties correctly. Periodic liver draining cures (for more see chapter 6), ideally taken at every change of the season, are therefore highly recommended.

The Intestines

The intestines form a tube approximately 7 meters (23 feet) long that originates in the stomach. They consist of two segments with different characteristics: the small intestine and the large intestine, or colon.

The small intestine measures anywhere from about 4 to 5.5 meters (13 to 18 feet) in length. It owes its name to the fact that its diameter is smaller than that of the large intestine: about 2.5 centimeters (1 inch) as compared to a diameter ranging from 5 to 6 centimeters (2 to 2½ inches). The first part of the small intestine is the duodenum. It is fixed in place and is the reception point for the digestive juices that are provided by the pancreas and the liver. The second part is mobile. It does not travel in a straight line but winds its way through the abdomen in numerous coils. The intestinal walls also release digestive juices. Working in tandem with those already present, they break down food into particles that are small enough to be absorbed by the body.

The majority of nutrients are absorbed in the lower part of the small intestine. This assimilation takes place at the level of the intestinal villi, which is the name for the thousands of tiny folds that carpet the insides of the intestine. Their role is to hold nutrients and increase the surface area for absorption. When the nutrients cross through the extremely thin walls of the mucous membranes, they enter the bloodstream, then the cells.

The walls of the intestinal mucous membranes are not only a path for assimilating nutrients but also a path for expelling substances from the body. Toxins that are being transported by the bloodstream can cross through the intestinal wall and be eliminated with the stools. This process of expelling undesirable substances from the bloodstream takes place along the entire digestive tract. The only visible signs of this process appear at the top of the tract: in the mouth. The white coating that can cover the tongue when an individual is suffering from a furred tongue consists of toxins that have been expelled. Because of the huge number of intestinal villi, the surface area of the small intestine is enormous. Hence its capacity for eliminating wastes is very

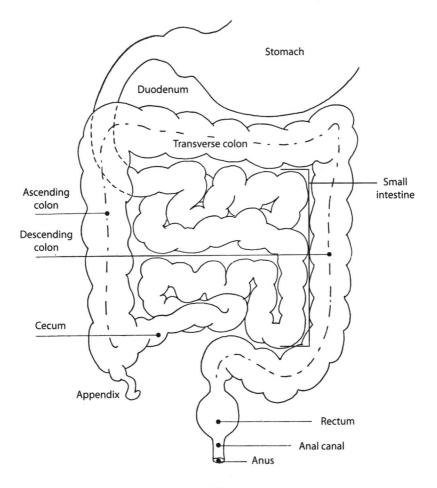

Fig. 3.2. The intestines

high. These wastes are characterized by a thick, soft consistency and the lack of a crystallized structure, meaning they are colloidal toxins.

The colon, or large intestine, has a diameter that averages about 5 to 6 centimeters (2 to 2½ inches) and measures around 1.5 meters (5 feet) in length. It originates in the lower right half of the abdomen around the level of the cecum. It climbs vertically along the right side of the abdomen then bridges it horizontally toward the left, just beneath the rib cage. It then goes back down vertically along the left side of the abdomen and forks toward the center of the body making an S shape that terminates at the anus.

Digestion and assimilation processes continue in the colon, but at the same time it is actively working to prepare wastes for elimination.

The process of elimination of wastes is active rather than passive. A veritable army of bacteria (the intestinal flora) attend to the transformation and preparation of wastes into a form that can be eliminated. Furthermore, the contraction of the intestinal muscles, known as intestinal peristalsis, is required to move these wastes toward the outer end of the intestines. Subtle mechanisms also come into play to ensure that enough water is retained in the stools to achieve a consistency that makes it possible for the body to evacuate them easily. If they lack water, they will be hard and dry. Their elimination will be difficult, and constipation will result. Conversely, when the stools are too liquid, they will not take any shape and will exit the body in the form of diarrhea.

🖐 Good to Know

Normally the intestines should empty one or two times a day. The speed of the intestinal transit should take twenty-four hours. For example, foods that we eat on Sunday should be leaving our bodies on Monday. We can monitor this speed by eating richly colored foods such as red beets or spinach. The pigments in these foods will color the stools red or green, respectively. The normal color of stools is brown.

The Stools

Stools are the support medium for the elimination of wastes through the intestines. They consist of approximately 80 percent water and 20 percent dry matter. This dry matter is primarily fiber or roughage, consisting of cellulose that because of its hard consistency has not been broken down enough by the intestinal flora. These fibers also contain the remains of dead germs and dead cells shed by the walls of the intestines. Stools are also made up of depleted minerals and proteins.

STOOLS AND WATER CONTENT

Lack of liquid	Constipation
Excess liquid	Diarrhea

Theoretically, there should be only a minimal amount of carbohydrates, fats, and proteins in the stools. These nutrients are supposed to be more or less entirely absorbed after having been prepared for assimilation by the digestive process. In practice, however, the digestive process is not always complete. This can occur when the digestive capacities are weakened and not up to the task of performing properly, or when the body ingests more food than the digestive capabilities can handle. In this event, poorly digested fats will remain in the intestines and the stools produced will be greasy. They will generally be lighter in color, even white, and will have a tendency to float. Poorly broken down starch can also be found in the stools. We should note in passing that both of these substances belong to the family of colloidal toxins.

? Did You Know?

According to some authors, one-third of the nutritive substances (starch, fat) we eat are not absorbed by the body and are eliminated with the stools.

In addition to the wastes that come directly from the foods we consume, we should consider those contained in the secretions of the digestive organs. These include, among other things, the wastes in the bile and all the wastes that have been processed for elimination by the intestinal walls, both of which are colloidal toxins.

The colloidal nature of intestinal eliminations is clearly demonstrated by a procedure intended to drain the colon: colonic irrigation. In this cleansing treatment a cannula (a small tube) with two openings is used. Water is introduced into the colon through one of these openings, and, when the colon is almost entirely filled with water, the now waste-laden water is allowed to pour out through the second opening.

This water flows through a transparent tube so the patient can see what is leaving the colon. These wastes often include gray or brown mucous clumps with a texture similar to egg whites; waste having a muddy, runny, and soft consistency; and yet another type that resembles rubber. Because these are all shapeless and non-crystalline, they are typical examples of colloidal toxins.

Breakdown of the Intestinal Filter

Normally, when the intestinal mucous membranes are in a healthy state, they allow only useful and fully digested nutritive substances to enter the bloodstream. The large molecules of poorly broken-down foods, such as residues of starch or fat, are forced to remain in the intestines where they can be evacuated by the colon. In theory, they are not assimilated and cannot overburden the body's internal cellular terrain. But this is only the case when the intestinal mucous membranes are in good condition. These membranes can often be damaged by toxins. The intestinal filter will then be partially destroyed, and the microlesions thus created will allow toxins to enter the bloodstream. The walls of the intestines become porous and no longer fulfill their role as a guardian of the internal environment of the body. The consequence of this is that toxins will enter and collect in the physiological terrain. The deterioration of the intestinal mucous membranes can also be caused by deficiencies in vitamin F as shown by Doctor Kousmine. Whatever the cause, the result is the same: the intestines cannot retain the toxins and they enter the bloodstream.

The causes of the partial destruction of the mucous membranes, and therefore the protective filter, are numerous. Regular consumption of irritating foods (spices, alcohol) can wound these membranes. Where overeating is an issue, the poison caused by the food substances fermenting and putrefying in the intestines can make them inflamed. Some food additives, medications, and gardening products (insecticides, herbicides) have the same effect. Even the stools can damage the mucous membranes when they remain in contact for too long, as is the case when the individual is constipated.

The Sebaceous Glands

The skin is richly scattered with about two million sebaceous glands. These glands are housed in the hair follicles, which is a fold on the skin surface out of which a hair grows. They can be found on almost the entire surface of the body except for the palms of the hands and the soles of the feet (both regions that are completely hairless). The strongest density of sebaceous glands is located on the face and scalp.

As an outgrowth of the follicles, the sebaceous glands are connected to them by tiny channels. These ducts secrete sebum, which contains a high proportion of fat—96 percent—as well as a variety of other colloidal wastes. Sebum's composition, therefore, is quite similar to that of bile. When it is still in the hair follicle, the sebum is fluid. It becomes semisolid when it reaches the skin surface. Here its role is to lubricate the skin, keeping it flexible and elastic. When too little sebum is released, the skin becomes dry and chapped. On the other hand, too much sebum will make the skin oily and greasy. An increase in the amount of the secretion is not due to a rise in the number of sebaceous glands but rather to an increase in their size. The cause can be hormonal, as is the case at the onset of adolescence. However, it can also be a defensive reaction of the body when there is an overlarge accumulation of colloidal wastes in the tissues. In

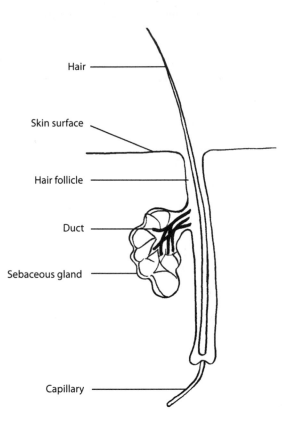

Fig. 3.3. The sebaceous glands

order to rid itself of some of these wastes, the body stimulates the sebaceous glands, which will then become overdeveloped (the medical term is *hypertrophied*) for a period of time.

When a sebaceous gland has become congested with sebum, it will produce a whitehead pimple. Oxidizing upon contact with the air, the sebum can harden and clog the pore. This pimple will be dark in color, earning its common name of blackhead. When the sebum is unable to leave the follicle it becomes stagnant. This will eventually create an inflammation and a small local infection. These conditions create the purulent red pimple typically associated with acne.

Each sebaceous gland secretes only a minute amount of sebum and, consequently, only a small amount of toxins. But, given the large number of these glands all over the body, the total quantity of wastes eliminated is substantial, especially since this elimination takes place continuously.

Sebum contains only a small amount of liquid so it is a support medium that is well suited to colloidal wastes. The high percentage of fat in sebum also indicates the colloidal nature of the wastes it transports.

The Lungs

The lungs are first and foremost a pathway for eliminating gaseous wastes; for example, the carbon dioxide we expel with every exhalation. But they can, when necessary, evacuate semisolid toxins. These wastes occur in the form of phlegm and spit, which are colloidal.

The toxins transported by the bloodstream come in contact with the lungs at the pulmonary alveoli. These are minuscule pouches that cluster together like grapes on a vine. Despite their tiny size, the entire expanse of their interior surfaces, if spread out, would cover 100 square meters (over 1,076 square feet), providing a huge surface for exchanges.

The blood capillaries that carry toxins into the lungs share a common wall with the alveoli. The wastes cross through this separating wall and find their way inside the alveoli. From there these wastes are transported through increasingly larger tubes (which diminish in number at the same time) to the body's surface.

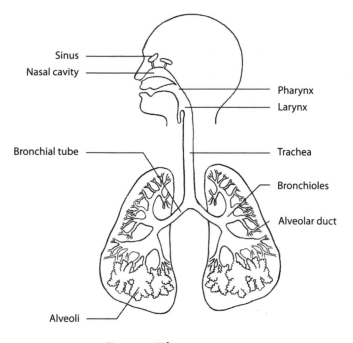

Sinus
Nasal cavity
Pharynx
Larynx
Bronchial tube
Trachea
Bronchioles
Alveolar duct
Alveoli

Fig. 3.4. The respiratory tract

In each lung, there are around thirty thousand tiny tubes called *bronchioles* or *bronchioli,* which drain the wastes collected by the alveoli. These bronchioles join together to form between fifty and eighty slightly larger conduits, the terminal bronchioles. These in turn combine to form five secondary bronchial tubes that then join together to form one bronchial tube. Because this occurs in each lung, there are two main bronchial tubes that meet at the trachea, which becomes the only path for the elimination of wastes. These wastes will eventually be expelled through either the nasal passages or the mouth, if coughing is involved.

The term *bronchial tree* is used when speaking of the

network of the lungs' bronchial tubes, because they continue to combine together until they form a common trunk resembling a tree with increasingly slender branches radiating outward. Wastes travel through this network from the tips of the branches to the trunk while at the same time the oxygen inhaled by the lungs travels in the opposite direction, from the trunk to the outermost tips of the branches.

It is easy to grasp how the contraction of the muscles can create a current that can carry something as light as carbon dioxide out of the body. But how are solid wastes, for example the dusts we inhale, and semisolid wastes like colloidal toxins, pushed to the exit?

The walls of the respiratory tubes are carpeted with a fringe of hairlike organelles known as *cilia* that move back and forth in the direction of the exit. Thanks to these movements, the cilia gradually carry and push forward dust and wastes. When these reach the bronchial tubes or the throat, they cause an uncomfortable sensation. The body then seeks to relieve this discomfort by violently expelling the wastes by coughing or spitting.

The sticky, runny nature of the wastes we blow from our noses, cough up, or expectorate classifies them without hesitation as colloidal wastes. Phlegm and other expectorants are clearly shapeless, flaccid, and lacking any crystalline or sharp properties.

> The wastes that we blow from our noses, cough up, or expectorate are colloidal substances.

Under normal circumstances, the mucous membranes of the alveoli allow only gases to pass through them (oxygen, carbon dioxide). However, when the bloodstream is overladen with toxins, they can also offer passage to wastes that are more cumbersome than gaseous molecules. The lungs then become an emergency exit for the elimination of colloidal wastes.

The colloidal wastes rejected by our lungs primarily come from the wastes produced when our diet is too rich or too abundant and exceeds the body's energy needs and digestive capabilities. But these wastes are also joined by the dead cells cast off by the respiratory tract, dead germs, and the protective mucus secreted by the mucous membranes of the respiratory tubes.

When an individual is enjoying good health, the respiratory tubes and nostrils will be entirely clear. The individual can breathe freely and easily, feeling no need to blow the nose or expectorate, unless having inhaled too much dust.

Conversely, respiratory tubes that have been pressed into service as an emergency exit for the elimination of colloidal toxins are overburdened and make breathing more difficult. Colloidal wastes are stagnating in the alveoli and bronchial tubes, or even in the nose and sinuses. When a person experiences shortness of breath due to physical effort, the wastes are displaced by the intensified back and forth movements of air causing the person to start spitting and expectorating. If individuals are severely clogged, they need only lean forward to allow these colloidal wastes to begin sliding out of the body: their nose will begin running.

THE ELIMINATORY ORGANS FOR CRYSTALLINE TOXINS

The Kidneys

We each have two kidneys. Located on either side of the spinal column, they are high enough to be protected by the bottom ribs. The wastes filtered through the kidneys are diluted in a liquid: urine. This urine is then conducted by a long tube—the ureter—into the bladder. There are two ureters; one for each kidney. When enough urine has collected in the bladder, the urge to urinate is signaled. The urethra then carries the urine out of the body.

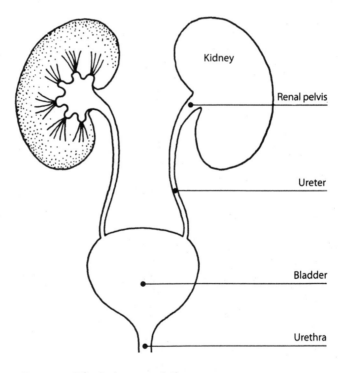

Fig. 3.5. The kidneys and the urinary tract

The kidneys are closely connected to the liquid element and thus to wastes soluble in liquid, like crystals. This fact clearly emerges when we study the way they function.

At about the size of a fist, the kidneys are quite small compared to the other organs and the entire body. However, they process more than a liter of blood per minute, which represents around a quarter of the amount of blood propelled into the vessels by the heart!

The kidneys function as a filter. This may be oversimplifying things, but we can say that the blood travels through this indispensable filter in two streams. On the one hand, we have the purified blood that continues to circulate through the blood vessels, and on the other, we have the waste-laden urine that will be eliminated from the body.

The basic filtration unit of the kidneys is the nephron, of which there are more than one million in each kidney. Tightly packed together, these nephrons form the outer shell of the kidneys. Each nephron consists of a glomerulus, which is the actual filter, and a tubule through which the urine produced by the kidney will flow. These nephrons are extremely tiny but perform a huge task all together.

Blood filtration, or the purification of the bloodstream by removal of its wastes, takes place as a result of the differing degrees of pressure that exists on either side of the glomerulus filters. Because the blood feeding into the glomerulus exerts more pressure on the filter than that with which it responds, a portion of this blood will be able to pass through the filter into the glomerulus. The filter of the glomerulus has a mesh with holes of a very specific diameter. They are too small to allow substances of large volume, such as red corpuscles or blood proteins, to pass through. However, smaller substances

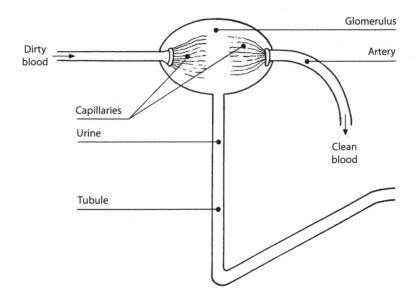

Fig. 3.6. The nephron

such as plasma (the liquid part of the blood), various minerals, urea, uric acid, creatinine, and so forth will be easily filtered into the glomerulus. These wastes belong to the crystal family.

Twenty percent of the blood that enters into contact with the glomerulus will be extracted and used to create urine for transporting the crystals. This filtration will create more urine than the kidneys will be able to eliminate though. In fact, glomerulus filtration produces 120 ml (4 ounces) of urine every minute, which amounts to around 180 liters in one day. This quantity is far higher than the 1.5 to 2 liters of urine eliminated on a daily basis. Before it is eliminated, urine undergoes a variety of transformations. The majority of the fluid part of urine is reabsorbed along with a number of mineral substances that are still useful to the body.

? **Did You Know?**

The necessity of sufficient blood pressure in order for this filtration process to work is illustrated by the fact that when blood pressure climbs, for example in situations where an individual feels fear, the person will feel a strong urge to urinate. This also explains why a beverage like coffee has a diuretic effect. The stimulating properties of coffee raise blood pressure. Blood pressure also rises during intense physical exercise or when swimming in cold water. Each time we see the same result: the need to urinate.

Conversely, when blood pressure is too low or if the heart is overly fatigued, urine production is weak. Not enough of the water taken in by the body is eliminated. This creates a risk of retaining water and developing edemas— the swelling caused by fluid retention in the body. This is especially visible in the ankles, which swell. The fingers will also increase in size, becoming noticeable when rings that were once easy to remove refuse to budge.

Every day we eliminate on average 1.5 liters of urine. This takes place over the course of five or six separate instances, as the urge to urinate will be felt when the bladder contains around 3 dl (10 ounces). This will vary from one person to the next, because the capacity to retain a large amount of urine is not uniform. Normal urine will have a lemon-yellow color and a characteristic odor.

☞ **Good to Know**

The reabsorption of liquid is based on the organism's water requirements. (For more on this see my book *The Water Prescription*.) When the hydration of the body is threatened, which happens when we do not ingest enough liquids, the amount of fluid available for making urine will be limited. Consequently, the volume of urine will be lower than normal, and its concentration will be quite high. While the body can forgo eliminating water, it does not have the same luxury when it comes to toxins. Consequently, toxins in the urine will increase dramatically in proportion to the smaller volume of urine. Their presence will make the urine darker; it will be deep yellow, or even brown, rather than a clear yellow. It will also have a strong odor. Urine can even be described as muddy when it has too high a concentration of wastes.

In the opposite situation, when an individual drinks more than necessary, there will be much more fluid available for manufacturing urine. The volume of urine will be greater, but its waste concentration will be proportionally lower. This urine will consequently have a very pale-yellow tint or even be transparent like water. Its odor will be much weaker, perhaps even nonexistent.

Urine is composed of 95 percent fluid. The remainder is crystalline waste: urea, uric acid, mineral salts, and so forth. The amount of urea that properly functioning kidneys can eliminate on a daily basis is about 15 grams on average. Depending on the individual diet (if one eats a lot of meat, for example), this quantity can double. Uric acid is eliminated at a rate of 0.5 to 1 gram per day. Unlike what occurs with urea, this quantity is relatively fixed. This means that the body has less flexibility when it comes to eliminating excess uric acid than it does with urea.

An insufficient flow of urine through the urinary tract has a harmful effect on the elimination of crystals. The risk is that the crystals that had dissolved in the urine will regain their crystalline state. This situation is vividly described by saying there is sand or grit in the urine. This sand will injure the mucous membranes of the urinary system. By combining into clusters, these crystals will form urinary or kidney stones. This normally occurs in areas like the kidneys or bladder, where urine lies stagnant for a period of time before being transported elsewhere.

> The formation of sand and stones, which can take place when the concentration of wastes in the urine is too high, shows how important a sufficient amount of water is to eliminating crystals.

The Sudoriferous Glands

Every square inch of our skin contains 70 to 120 sudoriferous (sweat) glands, which total about two million of these glands in the skin surface of the body.

Sudoriferous glands and nephrons function similarly. They both eliminate wastes with the help of a liquid support medium, sweat in this instance, and they both eliminate crystal wastes. The many striking similarities between the

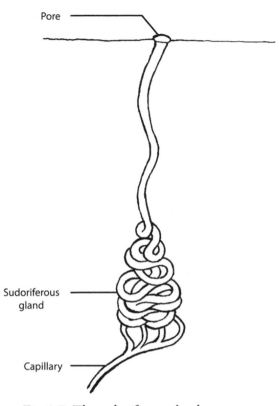

Fig. 3.7. The sudoriferous glands

sweat glands and the nephron often cause the sweat glands to be described as nephrons at skin level.

The filtering unit of the sudoriferous glands is also a glomerulus. This filter is located deep in the layers of the skin. As in the nephron, blood purification is a product of the pressures exerted on either side of the glomerulus filter. The pressure outside the glomerulus, where the blood is coming in, is higher than the pressure exerted inside the gland. This results in a portion of the fluid in the blood passing through into the glomerulus. Within this water are wastes of a very specific nature. In fact, the walls of the glomerulus act like a selective filter that, due to the size of its mesh, only allows certain substances to pass through. These are first and foremost crystals: urea, uric acid, and various minerals (such as sodium).

The liquid filtered by the sudoriferous glands, in combination with solid wastes, forms sweat. This sweat is carried along by a tube whose exit, on the skin surface, forms a pore. The sudoriferous glands are passive filters. They produce nothing on their own but work solely according to the pressure exerted on them by the bloodstream. The greater this pressure, the greater the irrigation experienced by the gland, and consequently the greater the amount of sweat it produces. This production is also dependent on heat. An increase in heat, and blood pressure, can have many causes. It can be the result of physical activity. It can also be due to the ambient temperature, the clothing we wear, taking a hot bath or sauna, a fever, and so forth. When the skin is cold, the circulation of blood at the level of the sudoriferous glands slows down immensely. This means the amount of sweat produced at these times is almost nil.

? Did You Know?

By sweat, we do not mean only the glistening drops that fall from the skin of someone who is perspiring heavily. In addition to this, the skin perspires throughout the day, which means tiny drops of water bead upon its surface. These evaporate instantly on contact with air, and for this reason, are not visible.

Perspiration by itself allows the elimination of 3 ml of sweat a minute, which amounts to 450 ml (about 15 ounces) in a twenty-four-hour period. The physical activities we inevitably engage in over the course of a day will cause more perspiration, which can range from 300 ml (about 10 ounces) to 1 liter a day. Accordingly, the body releases between 0.5 to 1.5 liters of sweat on a daily basis. This volume will increase even more if the individual engages in intense physical exercise. One session in the sauna will provide even stronger results. It is not unusual for a person to eliminate 1.2 liters of sweat in three ten-minute sessions in the sauna.

Emotion and stress are also factors to be considered. The release of adrenaline will raise blood pressure, and thus the pressure necessary for the sweat glands to filter.

Many people in today's world have a sedentary lifestyle. The quantity of crystal wastes they eliminate through their skin is therefore extremely small.

The crystal toxins eliminated by the sudoriferous glands require a liquid support medium to be transported outside of the body. Sweat has a 99 percent water composition. The remaining 1 percent consists of urea, uric acid, and depleted or excess mineral salts such as potassium, chlorine, and sodium.

> Sweat consists of 99 percent water as compared to the 95 percent of water in urine.

The amount of sweat eliminated depends not only on the blood flowing into the sudoriferous gland but also on the body's overall state of hydration. The elimination of sweat will be inhibited when a person drinks infrequently and the tissues experience a lack of liquid. When more liquid is consumed, there will be more sweat. The daily consumption of liquid necessary to remain in good health is approximately 2.5 liters daily.

CONCLUSION

The two different kinds of toxins—crystal and colloidal—are removed from the body by different eliminatory organs based on their solubility. Crystals are eliminated in a liquid support medium by the kidneys and the sudoriferous (sweat) glands; colloidal toxins are eliminated without the help of any support liquid by the liver, the intestines, the sebaceous glands, and the lungs.

4

The Different Illnesses Caused by Colloidal and Crystalline Toxins

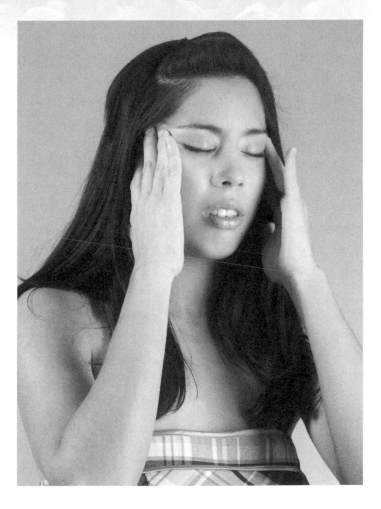

ℬ

Simply knowing that diseases are primarily due to the accumulation of toxins in the body is worthwhile, rather than remaining uninformed. However, it is even better to know how to tell the difference between those diseases that are caused by colloidal toxins and those created by crystalline toxins.

But how are we to proceed?

The first way of doing this is to observe which eliminatory organ, if any, is affected by the disease. As we have just seen, colloidal wastes and crystals do not use the same organs for exiting the body. Overloads of one kind of waste will target very specific organs. The other eliminatory organs will be spared completely, because they do not handle the waste products in question. For example, an excess of colloidal wastes can overwork and make several of the eliminatory organs that handle these toxins sick: the liver, intestines, lungs, or sebaceous glands. But the effects of this overload will have no bearing whatsoever on the organs that eliminate crystalline wastes from the body: the kidneys and sudoriferous glands.

> Colloidal wastes and crystals do not use the same eliminatory organs to exit the body.

This is why, when the liver, intestines, respiratory tract, or sebaceous glands are afflicted, we see evidence of a colloidal disease, because these organs specialize in the elimination of colloidal wastes. When the kidneys or sudoriferous glands are suffering from illness, we see signs of diseases caused by crystalline wastes, because these are the organs that are intended to eliminate crystals from the body.

The second way to tell what kind of illness—colloidal or crystalline—is present, and this is effective whether or not the disease has targeted a specific eliminatory organ, involves observing two symptoms: discharge and pain.

Colloidal Illnesses	Crystalline Illnesses
Discharge	No discharge
No pain	Pain

Colloidal illnesses cause discharges but do not hurt, whereas the diseases caused by crystals cause pain but have no discharge. This should be taken as a general rule and is not absolute as exceptions do exist.

THE DISCHARGE FACTOR

Some diseases are characterized by a visible discharge of substances from the body while others are not. The first are illnesses caused by colloidal wastes, the second are caused by crystals.

Colloidal wastes contain a certain amount of water, which gives them a semifluid consistency. Because of this they can overflow and be discharged once they reach a size that makes them visible to the naked eye. Colloidal wastes are discharged from the body by the respiratory tract (phlegm from colds, bronchitis, and so on), by the sebaceous glands (whiteheads, oozing eczema, varicose ulcers), and the intestines (in the stools).

It is true, however, that in some colloidal illnesses these wastes are present but do not cause discharges and therefore remain invisible. Among these exceptions to the general rule are cases of heaviness in the legs brought about by hemogliasis and cysts.

Crystals are basically hard, dry wastes with practically no water content. Consequently they do not flow or leave the body in the form of discharge. Instead they remain stationary, motionless. When there is an excess of crystalline waste in the body, they form deposits in the tissues. For example, these deposits can appear in the joints (arthritis), in the skin (eczema), on the walls of the blood vessels (arteriosclerosis), or in the kidneys' glomerulus (kidney stones). These deposits are extremely small in size, much smaller than the average collection of colloidal wastes, and are therefore much harder to see.

THE PAIN FACTOR

Pain is the result of an attack on the tissues. This assault can be either mechanical or chemical in nature. Crystals, as noted above, are hard and have an angular structure with sharp edges. When an excess of crystal toxins exists, they will compress the tissues, chafe against them, or outright injure them. When they remain stagnant in the body, they easily injure the cells by scratching, pricking, cutting, and piercing them, even causing ulcerations. Initially there will be an irritation, but over time lesions will occur. This inflammation makes the tissues extremely sensitive and all the more receptive to pain. A chemical assault is not caused by the physical presence of the attacker—its placement in the body or the pressure it causes—but by the actions of the chemical substances making up the toxin. Many crystals are, in fact, acids: uric, pyruvic, and so forth. These acids have a corrosive, burning, destructive, and ulcer-causing effect, as so many poisons and toxins do.

Conversely, colloidal wastes do not possess such attributes and do not cause pain. Their lack of structure, or rigidity, sharply reduces the possibility of attack. Being soft and malleable, they do not change the shape of the tissues they contact and do not tear or injure them like crystals. Instead, they change shape to adapt to that of their environment. It is difficult for them to maintain any kind of sustained pressure, because they are easily scattered and dispersed under pressure. Nor are their constituent elements aggressive or irritating.

🖐 Good to Know

We should point out that there are shades of gray when citing the lack of pain as a defining characteristic of colloidal diseases. A somewhat painful sensation will be displayed in some diseases such as bronchitis, for example. However, this pain is not as sharp, and most importantly not as continuous, as in the case of crystal diseases. The pains associated with colloidal diseases are due more to the inflammation caused by germs than toxins.

Now that we have established the general criteria that make it possible to tell the difference between the diseases caused by crystals and those caused by colloidal wastes, we can describe the different diseases to show their colloidal or crystalline properties in more detail. The question of mixed illnesses will also be discussed. In fact, the clogging of the terrain can sometimes be dual—involving both colloidal and crystalline toxins—which explains those illnesses that share characteristics of both kinds of diseases.

COLLOIDAL ILLNESSES

Respiratory Tract

Illnesses affecting the respiratory tract are typical of colloidal diseases. We shall start our examination of these diseases at the top of the respiratory tract and proceed down from there into the depths of the lungs.

Colds

The Greek word *rheuma,* from which the terms *rheumatic* and *rhume* (the French word for colds) are derived, means "flow." Another once common word for colds is *catarrh,* meaning "a heavy flow" or "discharge." The part of the body involved here is the upper end of the respiratory tract: the nasal cavities and the tubes leading into them. At the onset of a cold, the discharge is clear. Then, over a period of one or two days, it thickens and turns yellowish. These secretions are partially composed of the protective mucus produced by the mucous membranes, together with dead germs, but also include colloidal wastes.

When the discharge is predominantly mucus, the flow is

more fluid. When colloid substances are in the majority, it becomes thicker. The quantity of wastes eliminated can be quite large, as shown by the number of tissues used during some colds. On its own, a cold is not a painful disease, except for the burning sensation caused by the inflammation of the mucous membranes.

Chronic Cold

Some individuals suffer from a chronic runny nose. Instead of stopping after a few days, the discharge continues on a more or less permanent basis, although the sufferer can enjoy a few breaks from this flow now and then. This discharge of colloidal toxins can be free-flowing or it can be nonexistent. Its absence does not mean that these kinds of waste are not there though. They are still present, but as a blockage in the upper respiratory tract causing the feeling of constantly having a stuffed nose.

☝ Good to Know

The intensity of the chronic cold will vary depending on the body's production of wastes. It increases in response to overeating, for example. A similar increase occurs when the functioning of the liver or intestines slows down and the respiratory tract has to pick up the slack in order to eliminate these excess colloidal toxins.

Sinusitis

The sinuses are air-filled cavities in the bones of the jaws and forehead. The purpose of these hollow spaces is to lessen the weight of the skull and to serve as resonance chambers for the voice. The sinuses are connected to the nose by narrow tubes. While air can travel through these tubes quite easily, the same is not true for colloidal wastes. These wastes can stagnate in the sinuses and clog them, providing a hospitable environment for infections. Sinus inflammation creates a feeling of heaviness and throbbing pain. It varies between phases during which the nose is clogged and others where there is a discharge of mucus.

Bronchitis

Bronchitis starts with a dry cough and hoarseness. Only a few sticky globs are expectorated. But the elimination of phlegm subsequently becomes more substantial, because the bronchial tubes and the bronchioles have collected wastes that need to be eliminated. These wastes are not solely the remains of the dead germs responsible for the infection and the mucus the body secreted to protect itself in response, as generally believed. These secretions also contain the colloidal wastes transported by the blood and transferred into the lungs at the pulmonary alveoli level.

In order for an infection to develop in the bronchial tree, it is not enough for germs to find their way there. The terrain must also be receptive, and it becomes so when colloidal wastes collect there and stagnate.

Bouts of bronchitis are not always infectious. Sometimes they are due to the accumulation of colloidal toxins. These wastes collect in the bronchial tubes—reducing the passage of air and destroying the cilia intended to push them outward. To fight against the discomfort caused by the presence of these wastes, the glands that secrete mucus to lubricate the bronchial tubes begin working more actively. These membranes eventually expand and produce that much more mucus, which is then added to the colloidal wastes. The resulting sputum is copious and expelled from the body in large globs. As is typical of colloidal substances, the expectoration is viscous and gelatinous in form, which causes a greasy, wet cough.

Asthma

The small bronchial tubes and bronchioles of an asthma sufferer are congested with wastes. During an asthma attack the muscles that govern the expansion and reduction of the diameter of these tubes momentarily spasm, block the free passage of air, and prevent exhalation. At this point the fresh, rich, oxygen-bearing air cannot enter the lungs because the used-up air laden with carbon dioxide has not yet been expelled. This temporary inability to inhale creates the feeling of suffocation and is followed by an emergency defensive reaction of the body: a violent coughing fit. Large quantities of wastes are then expectorated, partially freeing the respiratory tubes. The spasm and coughing process is repeated several times. Between each attack the breathing is accompanied by a whistling noise caused by the forced introduction of air into channels that are too narrow, being clogged by colloidal wastes.

☞ Good to Know

Currently asthma is generally considered to be an allergic reaction. Often, though, no allergen can be detected. In fact, many asthma attacks are triggered by overly generous meals. The rate of excess colloidal wastes rises too sharply and burdens the lungs, causing the body to adopt defensive actions. The paramount role of colloidal toxins in the onset of these attacks is underscored by the fact that a strictly regulated diet, combined with stimulation of the organs that eliminate colloidal wastes such as the liver and intestines, will relieve or even banish these attacks.

The above description applies to wet asthma, the most commonly occurring form. A variant exists though—dry asthma—during which secretions are minimal. This asthma is a crystalline and allergic asthma. The spasms in this case are primarily due to the irritation caused by the crystals and allergens.

Skin

As with the respiratory tract, many ailments affecting the skin are primarily colloidal in nature.

Greasy Skin

The sebaceous glands release sebum to lubricate the skin. However, this secretion can be too abundant for some individuals, making their skin greasy and shiny. Adolescents, undergoing a stage when the work of the sebaceous glands intensifies, are most prone to this. Adults can also have greasy skin depending on the skin type of the individual and the quantity of excessive colloidal substances.

Whitehead Pimples

Pimples with whiteheads form over the sebaceous glands. They can be distinguished from crystal-caused pimples, which are large and red, located over the sudoriferous glands. In order for whiteheads to appear, a generous production of sebum is necessary as is the poor elimination of that sebum. Instead of freely exiting as it is produced, it stagnates and the gland becomes congested. This gland then becomes inflamed and creates a soft pimple with a whitehead. Such pimples frequently appear after dietary overindulgence: large meals, chocolate, pastries, and other foods that produce large amounts of colloidal wastes.

? Did You Know?

Pimples are the sign that the body in general and the liver in particular are being overburdened by the wastes they are receiving. When these wastes cannot be eliminated by the normal routes (liver, intestines), they will be conducted by a secondary emergency route: the sebaceous glands.

Oozing Eczema

Oozing eczema is defined as a "catarrhal inflammation of the skin," emphasizing the discharge (the catarrh) that is the typical characteristic of the diseases caused by colloidal toxins. This is an attempt by the body to get rid of an excess of these colloidal wastes. The work of the sebaceous glands is intensified, leading to an inflamed state. The filtration of wastes increases, and the abundant release of colloidal substances that ensues forms part of this discharge. The skin becomes red and swells due to small blisters that form along the tube that connects the sebaceous gland to the outside. The blisters, which provide another route for elimination, fill with a thick liquid that is largely colloidal and then burst. The skin oozes with this fluid and the wastes it contains, added to the wastes from the filtration process. This fluid then forms a crust as it dries.

Acne

The hormonal changes that take place during adolescence intensify the work of the sebaceous glands. Often this causes an excessively high production of sebum. This excess sebum then causes congestion in the gland, which becomes clogged and hinders its elimination from the body. Despite this, the body continues producing sebum, and as it accumulates it expands in size around and beneath the pimple. From the surface the sebum that is normally clear in color oxidizes and turns black. This dark spot is commonly known as a blackhead. When you squeeze it between two fingers, the pimple pops and releases a small streak of sebum that resembles a tiny noodle. This substance has a relatively soft consistency with nothing crystalline about it, which clearly identifies its colloidal nature. The area between several pimples can also become inflamed, which will then appear as a reddish purple patch on the skin. The pimples caused by acne become even more unsightly when infected.

🖐 Good to Know

An eruption of acne pimples is often stimulated by foods that produce colloidal wastes, such as bread, cookies, pastries, chocolate, and fatty foods like chips and fries.

Boil

The sebaceous glands are located in the hair follicles. When these follicles fill with too much sebum they create a terrain that is favorable to germs, especially the *Staphylococcus aureus*. When these bacteria multiply they create an infection that inflames the hair follicle. As the follicle gets more swollen and congested, it forms a large pimple that becomes increasingly painful. The pain is only temporary and vanishes as soon as the boil is popped to allow the pus to be released.

Carbuncle

When several boils next to one another merge together, they form a pus-filled area called a carbuncle.

Sty

A sty is a boil that forms on a follicle in the eye lid.

Sebaceous Cyst

Cysts are small sacs with rounded walls that form in different parts of the body. Their walls are tough. As their name indicates, sebaceous cysts are filled with sebum. This sebum can also contain other fluids or pasty materials. Cysts are like garbage cans filled with wastes, specifically colloidal wastes. They are sometimes open and either shrink or grow in proportion to how greatly the physiological terrain is overloaded. Others are closed and fixed in size. While it is possible to get rid of open cysts by draining them, this is not possible with the closed variety.

Circulatory System

The many afflictions to the circulatory system caused by colloidal toxins appear throughout the body from the blood vessels, to fat cells, and even to major organs such as the heart and brain.

Hemogliasis

Hemogliasis is a word mainly used in natural medicine. It means "thick blood." The loss of blood fluidity this condition implies results in slowed circulation. The oxygenation of the tissues is reduced. The heart has to pump harder to maintain circulation, and blood pressure rises. This disorder is quite common today. Doctors often prescribe blood thinners to fight against the increased viscosity of the blood.

☞ Good to Know

This thickening of the blood is due primarily to overindulgence in carbohydrates (grains, pasta, bread) and fats; both are food groups that produce colloidal wastes.

Varicose Veins

This is deformation of the veins, generally in the lower limbs, due to an accumulation of blood. The pressure the blood imposes on the vein walls causes them to dilate. They become deformed and twisted. This phenomenon can be seen easily when the veins are near the surface. Varicose veins are accompanied by a sensation of heaviness in the legs, sometimes accompanied by itching. The poor circulation that is the basis for varicose veins is caused by blood that is too thick, which makes it difficult to flow upward toward the heart.

Hemorrhoids

These are varicose veins in the region of the anus. They are also caused by overly thick blood. The colloidal nature of this disorder is given added emphasis by its connection to the liver, the organ charged with the duty of eliminating colloidal wastes. The veins in the anus are connected to the portal vein, which goes to the liver. When this organ is congested with wastes, the venous blood transported by the portal vein cannot flow freely through the liver and back into general circulation. This blood accumulates there, and its mass puts pressure on the vessels. The most vulnerable part of these vessels, the veins of the anus, suffers the consequences.

Arteriosclerosis

When colloidal substances—fats and cholesterol—are overly concentrated in the bloodstream, they cannot all be filtered from the blood by the liver. Some of them will form deposits on the walls of the blood vessels. There they form atheromas, or yellowish lumpy deposits. These deposits will grow larger and more extensive if they continue to be supplied with the colloidal wastes that formed them. In reaction to the presence of these foreign bodies a fibrous tissue is formed. This causes the vessels to lose their flexibility (sclerosis). With the accumulation of these deposits and the increase of this fibrous tissue, the diameter of the vessel becomes gradually smaller. The blood flow is obstructed. This in turn means that the organs irrigated by these vessels receive less and less blood. Arteriosclerosis is not painful on its own. It only starts to hurt when a vessel becomes very briefly clogged. In the heart area this translates into angina pectoris; in the calves it reveals its presence through intermittent cramping pain, which impairs walking.

High Blood Pressure

Blood that is too thick will have difficulty circulating, making the bloodstream flow more slowly. In addition, this will cause the organs (kidneys, liver) traversed by these blood vessels to become overburdened with wastes, just as the vessels themselves (atheroma). All of these factors combine to hamper blood circulation even more. In reaction to this situation, the heart increases the force it uses to circulate the blood. This inevitably results in a rise in blood pressure.

Heart Attack and Stroke

The blood can eventually become so thick that it coagulates and forms a clot. This clot can clog a vessel completely, which causes an interruption in the blood supply to the area of tissue dependent on the vessel. Once the supply stops, the tissue dies. This is particularly dangerous when this tissue belongs to a vital organ like the heart (heart attack) or the brain (stroke). These diseases are the culmination of a long process of blood being made thicker and thicker by wastes and the resulting overall deterioration of the vessels. Here, colloidal substances are no longer the only ones at fault. Crystalline wastes have combined with them. Together, they lead to a loss of blood fluidity.

Cellulitis

The body has adipose tissues that specialize in the storage of fats. These tissues are more highly developed in women than men, because they need to have larger fat reserves in the event of pregnancy. The basic element of these tissues is a fat cell called an *adipocyte*. These cells have the ability to store fats then release them when necessary. They are like small sacs that can fill and empty in accordance with the body's needs.

For various reasons (diet, hormones, a sedentary lifestyle), adipocytes can have enormous demand placed on them to store fats but little or no demand to release these stores. This will cause them to swell. They can swell to sixty times their normal size. When this happens, these swollen sacs are pushed toward the surface of the body in the form of bumps and pits on the skin. The substances they store are fats—elements of the colloidal family.

CRYSTAL DISEASES

Just as the eliminatory organs can be afflicted with conditions resulting from colloidal toxins, they can also be subjected to disease caused by crystal toxins.

Skin

Normally the sweat released by the sudoriferous glands is not concentrated enough to cause any damage to the skin. Skin disorders occur when it does become too concentrated. They can also appear when the skin does not perspire sufficiently and, consequently, becomes congested with the wastes that it should have eliminated.

Red Pimples

When the crystals eliminated by sweat are too high in number, they cause congestion in the sudoriferous glands. The pores of the skin become clogged. A collection of crystals gathers together and takes the form of a red pimple, which is hard and more or less painful. Unlike the pimples formed by colloidal substances, it discharges nothing. If you squeeze one with your fingers, nothing will come out.

Itching

When perspiration that is overloaded with crystalline and acidic substances spreads over the skin, it will irritate it. This attack is responsible for an itching sensation. This sensation can be more or less severe, depending on the case. Although it is not precisely a pain, which is one of the defining characteristics of crystal illnesses, it can come quite close.

Itching accompanies various skin disorders that are crystalline in nature: dry eczema, hives, allergies, and so forth. It can even appear by itself in the absence of any obvious disorder. Itching often occurs when an individual who rarely sweats suddenly begins perspiring heavily, for example, after strenuous physical exertion. The sudoriferous glands that are saturated with crystalline wastes will spill a very acidic sweat on the skin. The irritation this causes produces itching.

☞ Good to Know

In cases like this, it is possible to correct the tendency to itch. The sudoriferous glands should be regularly cleansed through voluntary sweating sessions: saunas, hot baths, and intense physical exercise.

Hives

An attack of hives is a prompt and efficient way for the body to rid itself of crystalline wastes. The skin becomes red and starts itching intensely. The appearance of the disorder appears suddenly and lasts for several hours. The most frequent cause is the consumption of certain foods such as crustaceans, pork, strawberries, eggs, and onions. This is not because the body is incapable of tolerating these foods; it is because they are rich in crystals and acids. When they are added to a cellular terrain that is already overburdened with wastes, they can cause the body's tolerance threshold to be surpassed. In a way they can be the final straw that breaks the camel's back—that last drop of water that causes the vase to overflow. This observation is supported by the fact that a lowering of the waste overload by drainings makes the attacks of hives disappear.

Dry Eczema

In dry eczema, areas of skin become red and dry under the corrosive effects of the crystals secreted by the sudoriferous glands. The skin gets so dry that it becomes cracked and chapped. This can be accompanied by a sensation of tension, burning, and itching. As its name indicates, this kind of eczema is not characterized by oozing and discharges. Being dry and connected with the sudoriferous glands, it is diametrically opposed to the wet eczema that is related to the sebaceous glands and colloidal wastes. Dry eczema can appear anywhere on the body but most often appears in those regions where perspiration is most intense, or where it is hard for sweat to evaporate. For example, this could include the regions beneath the armpits, between the legs, behind the knees, beneath the wristband of a watch, and so forth.

Chapped and Cracked Skin

Acidic sweat, perspiration that has a high crystal content, dries out the skin. The skin can lose so much of its suppleness that it starts cracking in spots. These cracks are often carved deeply in the skin with red walls and base. Because the skin is so sharply exposed this way it causes a certain amount of pain. The skin will be made even more fragile if is also under attack from inside by the crystalline wastes saturating the cellular terrain.

Herpes

The herpes virus is a common guest of the human body. It is only harmful when the internal cellular terrain allows it to multiply, which happens when the terrain is oversaturated with acids and crystals. Stress and intense emotions are also triggers, as they can acidify the terrain and lower the body's defenses.

Most often this infection affects the lips or nose. A red patch appears first and is soon followed by a tingling sensation. The patch becomes swollen and blisters appear, accompanied by a mild pain. Eventually these blisters burst. They release a little fluid that forms a crust. A wound that is sensitive to the touch will persist for several days.

Shingles

Shingles is a viral skin infection that develops in an acidic terrain saturated with crystalline wastes. In this disorder, small blisters with a bright red base form over the skin. They follow the trajectory of a sensitive nerve, which is why very intense pain is felt by individuals suffering from this disease.

Joints

It is not only the eliminatory organs that are adversely affected by the presence of crystal toxins. The joints of the body are susceptible to damage caused by a buildup of crystal wastes.

Arthritis

Arthritis is a typically crystalline ailment, meaning that it is an illness that is painful and without any form of discharge. Arthritis will not appear if crystal wastes are regularly and completely eliminated by the body as they are produced. But far too often the exact opposite is the case. The crystal wastes are poorly eliminated and start stagnating in the joints. The joints gradually deteriorate under the attack of these crystalline substances.

In allopathic medicine, arthritis is considered to be the result of natural wear and tear on the joints imposed by movement. But this wear and tear is primarily due to the presence of crystals. If wear and tear alone was the cause of arthritis, every elderly person should be stricken by it, especially those who were quite physically active in their younger days, which is not at all the case.

> The fundamental cause of arthritis is not natural wear and tear; it is the overconsumption of crystal-producing foods combined with weakness in the organs intended to eliminate crystalline wastes. Most often the kidneys are sluggish and the skin, because of a sedentary lifestyle, rarely or never perspires.

The headquarters for arthritis is the joint. A joint in the body is not a simple mechanical hinge that functions differently from the body's organs. A joint, like any other organ, is made up of cells that are nourished by the blood vessels. The cells for the various parts of the joint (bone, cartilage, tendons, sheath) are therefore equally dependent on the state of the physiological terrain. If the composition of this terrain is not good, their functioning will be disrupted and lesions will appear.

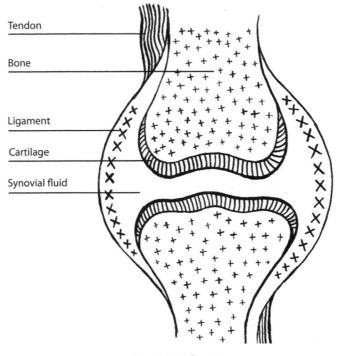

Tendon

Bone

Ligament

Cartilage

Synovial fluid

Fig. 4.1. The joint

Crystals can easily accumulate inside a joint. A joint acts as a gully where the blood vessels are narrower. This situation is similar to a river in that the wastes are less likely to be deposited when water flows through the large valleys than in the narrow gorges that form when the valleys shrink.

There are many different forms of arthritis, depending on the joint that is affected and how deeply it is stricken. But they can be broken down into three main groups representative of the three major stages of the progression in which crystals attack and destroy the joints.

> Crystals can easily accumulate inside a joint.

Arthritis Stage 1: The Isolated Arthritis Attack

The first manifestation of too many crystal wastes in the joints is an acute attack of arthritis. One of the joints will suddenly become inflamed. It becomes swollen, red, and extremely painful. At this stage it is generally the joints of the body's extremities that are affected, such as the hands and feet. Given the fact that the crystal invasion is only at its very beginning, this stage primarily affects young adults. The attack is temporary and only affects a single joint. If lesions persist, they are usually quite mild. This is the body's first warning that the continuous overload of crystals needs to be addressed. If nothing is done, the situation deteriorates and we move into stage 2.

Arthritis Stage 2:
Repeated Attacks of Chronic Arthritis

Here the attacks of inflammation repeat on a regular basis and with heightened frequency. The disorder becomes chronic because new crystals continue to arrive in the joints to combine with those already there. The overload rate is therefore much higher than in stage 1.

The joints that are now affected are no longer the small ones at the body's extremities but the larger ones closer to the center: knees, hips, neck, shoulders, and spine. The pains are now much more intense and the joint capsules become red and swollen. At this stage, several joints are generally affected. Because of the repeated nature of the attacks and because, even between these flare-ups, new crystals continue to arrive and attack the joints, the disorder ceases to be merely functional and begins to affect the structure of the joint. Every attack leaves repercussions in its wake. They reduce the scope of the joints' ability to open so the movement of the limbs is restricted. This restriction, in turn, means that the muscles involved get less use and begin to atrophy.

Among these aftereffects we should also include the deterioration of the cartilage in the joint. The ends of the two bones facing each other in the joints are covered in a smooth, shiny white cartilage. This allows the two pieces of bone to glide easily against each other when moving. This cartilage also serves as a buffer. Its flexibility and toughness allow it to absorb shocks. There is also a viscous fluid in the space that separates the two cartilages (and thus the two bones): the synovial fluid. This facilitates the sliding of the two surfaces against one another when demands are placed upon the joint.

The cartilage and the synovial fluid are the two key pieces in the construction of the joint. As it happens, both fall victim to an attack from crystals. Crystals, by virtue of their rugged surfaces, grate and scratch, and eventually wound the cartilage, making its surface rough. Crystals are predominantly made up of acidic substances. To neutralize these acids and prevent the damage they can cause, the cartilage will release alkaline minerals. This demineralization will cause it to weaken. Cartilage is also the part of the body that secretes synovial fluid. Its production of this essential fluid will also be reduced. The mechanics of the joint will no longer be as well lubricated. The result is that movement brings two worn-out, rough cartilages into contact, no longer separated by any synovial fluid. The deterioration of the cartilage by wastes is now accompanied by the wear and tear caused by every movement. Over time, the cartilage will vanish and the two naked bones are left facing each other.

☝ Good to Know

Normally, in a healthy body, movement does not cause any wear or tear because by stimulating blood circulation and cellular exchanges, movement actually regenerates the cartilage. It is only when the cellular terrain has been overladen with wastes that the cartilage deteriorates and movement becomes harmful to the joint.

The demineralization caused by acidosis not only affects the cartilage, it also harms the bones themselves. Bones are rich in calcium, an alkaline mineral that is used to neutralize acids. The muscles and tendons do not escape this harmful influence either. The consequence of their becoming weak and slack is that the two bones within the joint are no longer properly supported. When this occurs in the hand, the finger bones no longer remain aligned. The fingers start leaning to one side or curling in on themselves.

When the body finds itself confronted with all these assaults, it does not remain a passive spectator. It tries to limit the damage to the maximum possible extent. One of the defense methods it implements is to strengthen the tissues that are under attack. In order to do this, it triggers a multiplication of cells that will cause the attacked tissues to grow thicker. This can occur either in the cartilage or the bone. This process (hyperplasia) reinforces the stricken part of the body. The drawback is that this increases the size of the tissues and makes them more fibrous in order to best resist friction. This becomes problematic because the components of the joint capsule will assume a shape that is not correct. These deformations hinder movement, which becomes restricted and difficult.

This process of deterioration becomes even more pronounced in the following stage.

Arthritis Stage 3: Osteoarthritis

Osteoarthritis is an arthritis that causes physical deformation, generally confined to a joint. This is the final stage that arthritis cases will inevitably reach if nothing is done to curb their development. Consequently, it is a form of arthritis primarily suffered by the elderly. Depending on its location in the body, it can have different names: gonarthrosis when in the knees, coxarthrosis when in the hips, spondyloarthritis when the spinal column is affected, and so on.

The corrosive effect of the acids and the injurious effect of the crystals lead to the shrinkage of the cartilage, which eventually will disappear. The bone then begins deteriorating. It is attacked by the acids and by the friction of movement. The presence of acids also sets in motion an attack from within by forcing the bone to surrender its minerals to neutralize the acidity.

The tissue changes described above are worsened by the deposit of depleted minerals, salts left by the neutralization of acids by alkaline substances, crystals, and other wastes on the bone surfaces. There they form nodules and growths that cause the bone to become more deformed and more greatly hinder movement.

In osteoarthritis the joint becomes stiff and inflexible. It will grate when moving, and its range of movement is restricted and painful.

☝ Good to Know

Arthritis is generally aggravated by changes in the weather. Cold temperatures and dampness are particularly hard to tolerate. Low temperatures slow down the cellular exchanges in the tissues, which increases the clogging of the joint capsule.

The first two stages of arthritis are inflammatory stages, characterized by heat. The chief characteristic of the third stage is cold. The inflammation is greatly reduced but the degeneration of the joint stealthily continues. Its progression is indicated more by the joint's diminished range of movement than by any inflammation.

Gout

Gout's characteristic trait is sudden, sharp pains, most often in the area of the big toe (but they can sometimes appear in the hands). The toe becomes swollen and shiny red and is extremely sensitive to touch. A fairly high fever can also appear. The inflammation of the joint is due to the presence of crystals (uric acid) coming from a diet rich in proteins (meat, deli products, seafood) or foods with acidic properties identifying them as crystal foods: wine, beer, coffee.

Kidneys

The kidneys are the exit route for the elimination of protein wastes (uric acid, urea), various acids, and expended minerals.

Kidney stones are the primary ailment that appears in this eliminatory organ due to the presence of an overabundance of crystalline wastes. When the quantity of crystals that need to be eliminated from the body is high but the quantity of water needed to produce urine is low, the crystals have a tendency to collect and form stones, or masses with a sharp, crystalline shape. They deposit in the renal cavities in the pelvis or in the bladder. There are several kinds of kidneys stones, including those made from calcium oxalates, urates, and phosphates. As long as the stones remain inside the cavities where they formed, they do not cause any major problem. Problems emerge primarily when they enter the ureter or urethra because the diameter of these tubes is sometimes too small to allow them to pass through easily. The result is extremely sharp pain.

Nerves and Muscle

As we saw with the joints, crystalline wastes and particularly the acids belonging to that group can have a very damaging effect on the nerves and muscles of the body.

Neuritis

Nerves that have been weakened by crystalline wastes will become inflamed when the acid burden increases. This often takes place upon considerable physical exertion, combined with a strong demand placed on the nerves by sudden, violent movements. When this occurs in the area of the elbow, it is called epicondylitis, or tennis elbow.

Tendonitis
This is a painful inflammation of the tendons caused by crystals.

A Tendency to Feel Stiff and Achy
Every physical effort produces lactic acid in the muscles, an acid that belongs to the family of crystalline wastes. This acid is poorly neutralized and eliminated by individuals leading a sedentary lifestyle. It will lie stagnant in the muscles causing them to feel stiff and achy.

SPECIAL CASES

Diseases of the Digestive Tract
The diseases of the digestive tract are a special type. The organs of the digestive tract are more often confronted by food than by toxins. Thus the illnesses they suffer from are more often due to difficulty in the digestion of food than to attacks from wastes. Having said this, it should be noted that crystal-producing foods cause illness of some organs and colloidal-producing foods affect others. Despite this it is still possible to divide digestive ailments into colloidal or crystalline diseases.

For example, proteins are primarily digested in the stomach and then in the colon, which makes these two organs vulnerable to disorders that are crystalline in nature. Starches and fats primarily put a demand on the liver and small intestine, so these two organs are subject to illnesses that are colloidal in nature.

Dental Cavities

When weakened by mineral loss caused by the acidification of the cellular terrain and by the aggressive presence of acids, teeth tend to form cavities. This causes pains but no discharge, the identifying traits of a crystal disease.

Canker Sores

Canker sores are small ulcers located on the mucous membranes of the mouth. They are caused by the corrosive effect of acidic substances. They are painful and produce no discharge.

Gastritis

Stomach inflammation and the pain it causes are not the direct result of crystals but of foods that produce them such as meats, delicatessen products, and so on. They create too heavy a demand for the stomach's acid secretions, which will then start attacking the mucous membranes of this organ.

Liver Weakness

Without causing any actual illness, the liver can be in a weakened state and working below its normal capacities. This will result in an insufficient quantity of the bile it produces, which will in turn create digestive disorders. These can include difficulties digesting fats and large meals, feelings of nausea, bloating, migraines, and so forth. This prompts a diagnosis of hepatic weakness or insufficiency, or even a sluggish liver.

The liver is the organ that makes the bile necessary to digest fats, which are producers of colloidal wastes. When there is an overabundance of fats or even simple overeating, the liver becomes fatigued and is unable to produce enough bile. Bile has the task of eliminating colloidal wastes from the body.

Intestinal Fermentation and Bloating

The small intestine is the part of the digestive tract where starches—grains, breads, pastas, cookies, and crackers—are digested. When the functioning of the small intestine is weak, foods that are rich in starches are poorly digested and begin to ferment. The result of this is a vast increase in the production of gas. This gas will distend the intestinal walls, which can feel like having a large ball in the belly. These problems are not due directly to colloidal toxins but to the foods that produce them.

Colitis

The colon is where proteins are digested. When the intestinal bacteria in the colon is unbalanced, the protein remnants from food begin to putrefy. This creates a number of poisons that attack the mucous membranes of the colon. The result is inflammation. It is painful because there is a constant introduction of newly chewed food (the bolus) that comes into contact with the now ultrasensitive walls of the colon. The connection with proteins and the presence of pain make colitis an illness with crystalline characteristics.

Colloidal–Crystal Combinations

What I have said until now can give the impression that not only the eliminatory organs but also all diseases are exclusively colloidal or crystalline. In reality, as I pointed out at the beginning of this chapter, this is not always the case. There are instances of a combination of crystalline and colloidal substances in diseases and in the eliminatory organs.

> There are instances of a combination of crystalline and colloidal substances in diseases and in the eliminatory organs.

At the start of any illness, there is generally one single eliminatory organ that is weakened and posing a problem. If, for example, it is an organ intended to eliminate colloidal wastes from the body, it will create colloidal diseases. Over time, however, a second organ can become weakened due to lifestyle, an accident, or any one of a number of reasons. In some cases this organ will be of a different type than the organ that was first afflicted.

What this means is that until the second organ became a problem, there was only one kind of waste that was accumulating in the cellular terrain; now though the terrain is becoming overburdened with both colloidal and crystalline toxins. The diseases that arise will sometimes belong to one of these types, sometimes the other. But the simultaneous presence of large amounts of colloidal wastes and crystalline wastes in the terrain can also, over the long term, lead to diseases that combine both types: crystal–colloidal diseases.

In these cases it is no longer just one kind of toxin that is responsible for the health disorders, but a combination of the two. Their shared presence means that their damage potential multiplies. Following are several examples.

Cardiovascular Diseases

Heart attacks, high blood pressure, arteriosclerosis, hemogliasis, and so forth are fundamentally colloidal diseases, which is to say illnesses caused by an excessive consumption of foods rich in fats and starches. But the people who tend to develop these diseases are also prone to overindulging in proteins, or meat, which is a large producer of crystals. In fact the atheroma plates that form on and within the blood vessel walls do not only consist of fats (colloidal substances). Crystal deposits are also appearing here. It is these crystals that are responsible for calcifying the vessels, which causes them to lose their elasticity and makes them brittle.

High blood pressure is generally due to blood that has become too thick because of an excess of colloidal toxins. But sometimes congestion of the kidneys by crystalline wastes also contributes. Both of these factors hinder the normal blood flow. The heart has to increase the force needed to propel blood into the vessels, hence the high blood pressure.

In a heart attack, the blood clot that clogs the coronary artery due to thickening of the blood, is generally caused by overeating. Colloidal and crystalline substances are therefore both present.

Degenerative Diseases

Cancer, multiple sclerosis, polyarthritis, and so on are all degenerative diseases. They are the final consequence of a long process of fouling and clogging the cellular terrain, which the body has been fighting to the best of its abilities. This is a progressive process that goes through several stages.

The first stage takes place when this clogging process begins. The body's vital forces are still powerful enough to create a cleansing crisis that will expel the bulk of the wastes that have been accumulated in the terrain. These crises occur in the form of acute, violent illnesses that are of short duration. However, if nothing is done to halt the clogging process, the body will tire and not react as forcefully as time goes by.

This brings us to the second stage of these diseases. The body is only able to eliminate a portion of these excess wastes and has to repeat these efforts over time. These repeated attempts to eliminate these accumulated wastes are the defining characteristic of chronic diseases. Until this stage the body's efforts have been centrifugal, meaning that the wastes were expelled toward the outside. This is evidence that the body still had some vital force at its disposal. Unfortunately, this force will diminish over time if no changes are made to the individual's diet and lifestyle. A time will come when the body is no longer capable of creating an eliminatory crisis.

This is when the centrifugal motion becomes transformed into a centripetal movement, meaning it is directed inward (the third stage). Toxins collect more and more inside the body. They no longer cause any damage when exiting the body as in the previous stages but remain stored within. Here they can inflame the tissues (polyarthritis, in which four or more joints are afflicted), destroy the tissues (multiple sclerosis), or cause them to mutate (cancer).

THE THREE STAGES OF CHRONIC DISEASE

Stage	Elimination Crises	Diseases	Movement
1	Violent and single cleansing of the bulk of toxins	Acute	Centrifugal
2	Weak and repeated, few toxins expelled	Chronic	Centrifugal
3	Absence of eliminatory crises	Degenerative	Centripetal

The severe clogging of the terrain, which is the primary cause for the body's degeneration, is both colloidal and crystalline in nature. In fact, it is the culmination of a fouling process that has extended over many years. The eliminatory organs that have been weakened by the deterioration of the terrain are, consequently, both those responsible for colloidal wastes and for crystalline wastes. Additionally, the root cause for this overload of toxins is generally overeating, an excess consumption of both colloidal and crystalline foods.

> The severe clogging of the terrain, which is the primary cause for the body's degeneration, comes from a mixture of both colloidal and crystalline wastes.

Constipation

Constipation is the term for the difficulty or impossibility of evacuating stools from the body because they are too hard and dry. In addition to a lack of fiber, the foods that contribute to this health disorder are both foods that produce colloidal wastes (by excessive consumption of fatty foods that exhaust the liver and reduce the production of bile, which has a lubricating effect on the intestines) and foods that create crystal wastes (by excessive consumption of proteins in general). The treatment of constipation calls for methods to fight against crystals (drink lots of water) and colloidal wastes (stimulate the liver).

Bile Stones

The bile that is stored in the gallbladder to be used during a large meal is intentionally concentrated to improve its effectiveness. This process of concentration can become too productive however. This occurs when the bile is overloaded with colloidal wastes or the walls of the gallbladder lose their tone. When the latter happens, their contractions will not be strong enough to expel sufficient amounts of bile. The bile then tends to stagnate, and the substances it had dissolved may begin to collect together. Deposits of cholesterol, biliary salts, and calcium salts will then form. Because of their connection to the hepatic system and their composition, bile stones are primarily colloidal wastes. But because of their mineral content and their hard, structured shape, they are crystalline in nature at the same time. Bile stones do not become a problem unless their number or size hampers the contraction of the gallbladder. They become dangerous when they enter the bile ducts. If they block these ducts, always a possibility, they will cause sharp pains and a risk of hepatitis.

Ringworm, Candida

The yeasts and fungi that live in our bodies are micro-organisms that feed on the wastes of proteins, fats, and carbohydrates. Because of this relationship a rapid growth of yeasts or fungi is only possible when the level of these toxins is high. The higher the levels of these toxins, the larger the population of the microorganisms that feed on them can be. Because of their mixed origin (proteins, fats, carbohydrates), the wastes they produce are also a mixture of crystals and colloidal substances.

> The proliferation of yeasts and fungi is only possible when the level of toxins is high.

Allergies, Hay Fever

In naturopathy we understand that (aside from an inherited predisposition) it is only when the cellular terrain is under heavy attack from toxins that the body—already on the defensive because of the quantity of toxins present—will block out a substance, reacting disproportionately to it in the future. This substance (which can be pollen, cat hair, dust, and so forth) is not the true culprit. The actual cause is the terrain that is already saturated with both colloidal and crystalline wastes (and weakened by nutrient deficiencies).

The Mixing of Toxins in the Eliminatory Organs

We have spoken with good reason of the various eliminatory organs as hepatic, renal, and intestinal filters. These organs actually function as if they possessed a mesh filter that selects what passes through them (toxins) and what is retained (nutritive substances, blood components, and so on). To be effective in their work, the mesh of the filter must be in good condition and must reflect the filter's specialty in dealing with colloidal or crystalline substances. Unfortunately, when a body has been overburdened with wastes for a long time, the filters will be injured and display lesions.

The wear and tear on the mesh by toxins causes them to gradually lose the ability to select what stays and what goes through. Instead of allowing only the wastes they specialize in eliminating to pass through—crystals or colloidal wastes— the organ now sometimes lets the other kind of wastes through. This results in a blended waste product traversing the organ. This is especially common in the respiratory tract. The respiratory tract is designed for the elimination of colloidal toxins. But excessive amounts of toxins and the wear and tear they inflict on the filters can force them, contrary to their initial design, to also expel crystals. This results in diseases that are crystalline in nature.

> The wear and tear on the mesh by toxins causes them to gradually lose their ability to select what stays and what goes through.

Dry Cough

The dry cough can be powerful but nothing is expectorated. The crystals in the respiratory tubes irritate them causing them to become painfully inflamed. What we see in these cases is pain without any discharge, the signature characteristic of crystal-caused diseases.

Dry Bronchitis

The customary inflammation and coughing is present, but practically no colloidal wastes are expectorated.

Dry Asthma

The flow of colloidal wastes are absent. If some colloidal matter is expectorated, examination of it will reveal gritty bits of waste: crystals.

An opposite example is the tear glands. These are glands that eliminate crystals in the tears. This is the sand we rub out of our eyes every morning when we awake. But following heavy meals, these deposits in our eyes can resemble colloidal substances rather than crystals.

CONCLUSION

Because of their different characteristics, colloidal wastes and crystalline wastes engender different diseases. Generally speaking, diseases that are the work of colloidal wastes are accompanied by discharges but no pain. The illnesses caused by crystals are painful but do not have any discharges.

5

Food Sources of Colloidal and Crystalline Toxins

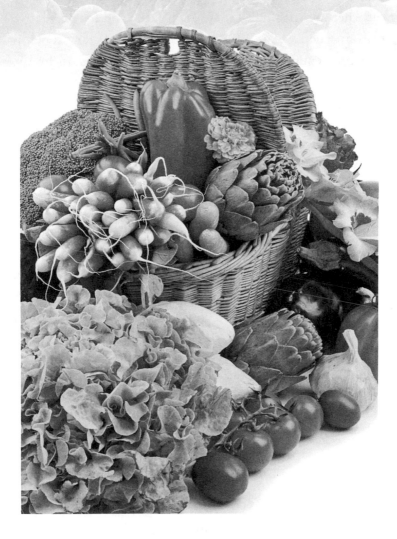

The origins of colloidal and crystal wastes are the foods we eat. It is therefore of fundamental importance to recognize which foods produce colloidal substances and which ones create crystals. This is how we can regulate the foods we eat when we wish to alleviate an ailment and for preventive reasons when we are in good health. This dietary supervision can reduce the clogging of the cellular terrain by the kinds of toxins that are responsible for health problems. For example, a person suffering from a disease caused by crystalline wastes can reduce the consumption of foods that produce crystals.

As we saw at the beginning of chapter 2, nutrients, proteins, carbohydrates, and fats all produce a specific kind of toxin. Proteins produce crystals while carbohydrates and fats produce colloidal wastes. Obviously, most foods consist of all three kinds of substances but in different proportions. It is rare for a food to be made up of only one of these substances, for example proteins. Generally, a substantial amount of a second kind of nutrient is also contained in the food, although

THE NUTRIENTS AND THEIR TOXINS

Nutrient	Kind of Toxin
Protein	Crystals
Carbohydrates	Colloidal substances
Fats	Colloidal substances

in lesser quantity than the principal nutrient. When the ratio of this secondary element is high, the primary toxin of the food will be combined with the other kind of toxin.

☝ Good to Know

Foods cannot always be definitively classified as the producers of only crystalline or colloidal wastes. It is not so black and white; there are many shades of gray. Some foods are primarily producers of one kind of waste and produce smaller quantities of the other kind.

We should stress the fact that just because a food produces lesser amounts of one kind of waste does not mean that the amount of that waste is small. This production can be just as high as a food that is a principal producer of the waste in question. For example, beans are a secondary producer of crystals, but this production (23 percent) is a bit higher than that of meat (20 percent), a primary producer of crystalline wastes.

PRIMARY PRODUCERS OF COLLOIDAL WASTES

Grains

Cereal grains (wheat, oats) are extremely high in carbohydrates. They contain between 50 percent and 80 percent. These carbohydrates occur in the form of starch, which consists of chains of more than ten thousand glucose molecules. These long chains need to be broken down into their constituent elements: single glucose molecules. When this does not take place, chains consisting of several dozen or even hundreds of glucose molecules remain. These chains form colloidal wastes. The higher the starch content of a grain, the more colloidal waste it will produce.

While grains have a high carbohydrate content, they also contain significant amounts of proteins. They are less in quantity than the carbohydrates but are still substantial. They are generally at levels of about 10 percent, which is about half that contained by meat (20 percent). This is why grains are primarily foods that produce colloidal wastes but are a secondary level producer of crystals.

Food	Carbohydrate Content Percentage	Protein Content Percentage
Flours		
Oats	65%	12%
Wheat	69.4%	12.1%
Buckwheat	70%	11.7%
Rye	72%	11%
Barley	72.3%	11.5%
Corn	76.1%	7.8%
Rice	78%	7.5%
Breads		
Brown bread	49%	9.3%
Whole wheat bread	50%	8.1%
Rye bread	51%	7%
White (wheat) bread	57%	6.9%

Food	Carbohydrate Content Percentage	Protein Content Percentage
Grain Products		
Spice bread	72%	8.5%
Wheat crackers	75.2%	9.9%
Wheat semolina	76%	10.3%
Pasta	76.5%	12.8%
Butter cookies	77%	5.6%
Tapioca	82%	1.5%
Rice flakes	87%	6.7%

Starchy Foods

Some foods, despite not being grains, are also very high in starch and thereby the producers of colloidal wastes.

Food	Carbohydrate Content Percentage
Potato	18.9%
Chestnut	42.8%

Cheeses

Aged cheeses, whether hard cheeses like Swiss or cheddar or soft in consistency like Brie or Camembert, are concentrated foods. Their high fat content makes them foods that produce colloidal wastes. Nonetheless, they contain a high amount of protein; in fact, they contain as much of this nutrient as meat. Therefore they are a secondary producer of crystalline wastes.

Food	Fat Content Percentage	Protein Content Percentage
Goat cheese	20%	20%
Brie	20.9%	17%
Camembert	23.9%	19.4%
Muenster	24%	21%
Parmesan	25.5%	38%
Monterey Jack	25.6%	24%
Cheddar	26.3%	24%
Provolone	28.8%	25%
Saint-Paulin	29%	24%
Mozzarella	29.4%	22%
Cantal	30%	23%
Gruyere/Swiss	30%	29%
Emmentaler	31.8%	27.7%
Roquefort	33.5%	22%
Blue Cheese	34%	24%

Oils and Fats

Vegetable oils, such as olive oil and sunflower oil, as well as concentrated fats (butter, lard, and other cooking fats) are not foods that occur naturally but are extracts and concentrates created by human beings. Their fat content is therefore quite high. It borders on 99.9 percent for vegetable oils, both those used for cooking and salad dressing. The concentration of animal products like butter or lard is a little lower but still quite high as can be seen in the following table. When they are not metabolized properly, these food products can produce substantial amounts of colloidal wastes.

Food	Fat Content Percentage
Of Vegetable Origin	
Coconut oil	98%
Vegetable oil	99.9% (olive, sunflower, etc.)
Of Animal Origin	
Cream	35%
Mayonnaise	39.5%
Fresh butter	81%
Margarine	83.5%
Lard	90.7%

It should be noted that virgin vegetable oils, whose first pressing is cold, contain more unsaturated fatty acids (easy to metabolize) than oils that are heat pressed. Consumption of large amounts of these oils will produce less colloidal waste than the heat-pressed oils. Cooking these oils at high heat will saturate these unsaturated fatty acids, which is the reason cooked fats cause greater amounts of colloidal waste than the oils that are used raw.

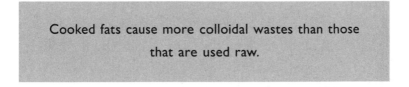

Cooked fats cause more colloidal wastes than those that are used raw.

Oleaginous Seeds and Nuts

As their name suggests, oleaginous foods are rich in oil, and therefore in fats. They have a lower protein content, but it can still be substantial. They are therefore primarily colloidal waste producers and secondary producers of crystalline wastes.

Food	Fat Content Percentage	Protein Content Percentage
Fresh black olives	15%	1.6%
Fresh green olives	20%	0.8%
Fresh coconut	34.5%	4.1%
Dried peanut	40%	23%
Cashew	48%	19%
Sunflower seed	50%	22.3%
Almond	54%	20%
Pistachio	54.5%	21.5%
Pine nut	60.4%	12.4%
Dried hazelnut	60.5%	13.3%
Dried walnut	62.2%	15% (plus a lot of acids)
Brazil nut	65%	15.1%

Beans

Beans like lentil and soy are known for their high nutritional value. Carbohydrates are the nutrient most highly concentrated in beans. Carbohydrates are present at a level of 30 percent to 60 percent, which makes beans a food that produces colloidal wastes. But beans are also extremely high in proteins, and this makes them a secondary producer of crystals. Their average protein content is around 23 percent, which is slightly higher than the protein content of meat (20 percent).

Soybeans are an exception to the rule. It is the richest source of proteins (35 percent) of all foods. Some beans also have a high content of purines, the precursors of uric acid, another crystalline waste.

Food	Carbohydrate Content Percentage	Protein Content Percentage
Soybean	29.9%	35%
Lentils	55.9%	24.5%
Dried peas	58.3%	23.8%
White beans	58.8%	20.2%
Chickpeas (garbanzo beans)	61%	18%

PRIMARY PRODUCERS OF CRYSTALLINE WASTES

Meats

This category includes red and white meats, poultry, game, treated meats like delicatessen cold cuts, fish, and seafood. These are foods that are high in proteins; their content of this nutrient, which is a producer of crystalline wastes, falls between 15 percent and 25 percent. They are also great producers of crystals for another reason. Because they are animal flesh—tissues consisting of numerous cells—these foods contain phosphoric and sulfuric acids. In fact, these acids are inevitably found in the core of every animal cell as they are an integral, constituent part of the proteins of the core. Both these mineral acids belong to the family of crystals. This is why cheeses, which are not tissues, do not contain these substances.

The table that follows provides the protein content of animal meats going from the lowest to the highest concentrations in each category. The greater the protein content in a food, the more crystal waste it will produce. All we are looking at here is the protein content. In fact, the quality of a kind of meat is not dependent on protein. Pork is not a better meat than rabbit just because pork contains less protein (16 percent) than rabbit (20 percent). Other factors come into play such as the fat content, for example, or the kind of food the animal was fed.

Food	Protein Content Percentage
Meat	
Lamb	16%
Pork	16%
Mutton	17%
Beef	18.2%
Veal	19.6%
Rabbit	20.4%
Fowl	
Duck	16%
Turkey	20.1%
Chicken	20.8%
Game	
Deer (buck)	20%
Wild boar	21%
Deer (doe)	21.4%
Hare	22.3%

Food	Protein Content Percentage
Processed Meats	
Hot dog	11.5%
Kielbasa	13.3%
Liver pâté	14%
Bratwurst	14.3%
Pepperoni	20.3%
Chitlins	23%
Salami	24%
Hard sausage	24%
Fish	
Cod	16.3%
Hake	17%
Mackerel	18.7%
Trout	19.2%
Salmon	19.9%
Fresh tuna	27%
Shellfish, Seafood	
Oysters	9%
Mussels	11.9%
Lobster	16.2%
Crab	16.9%
Shrimp	18.7%
Scallops	26.3%
Clams	29%

Some animal meats are also high in fat. This rate is sometimes higher than that of protein, which technically makes them primary producers of *colloidal* wastes—though they are still *very* significant producers of crystalline wastes and have been categorized here with the rest of the meats for simplicity. This is the case for the following foods.

Food	Fat Content Percentage	Protein Content Percentage
Meat		
Mutton	18.7%	17%
Lamb	24%	16%
Pork	25.2%	16%
Rack of pork	30%	15%
Lamb chop	30%	15%
Mutton chop	32%	14.9%
Fowl		
Duck	28.6%	16%
Goose	32.5%	16.2%
Processed Meats		
Cooked ham	20.6%	19.5%
Cured ham	30.5%	15.1%
Salami	35%	24%
Sausage	38%	14%
Blood sausage	41%	28%
Liver pâté	42%	14%
Hard sausage	51%	25%

☞ **Good to Know**

Protein foods that are low fat or have a fat content lower than their protein content are beef, veal, rabbit, game meats, fish, and seafood. These foods can be considered to be exclusively crystal producers.

Some Dairy Products

Soft white cheeses and yogurts are foods that are primarily crystal-waste producers and secondarily colloidal-waste producers, whereas the opposite is true for all other dairy products (cf. cheeses on page 112). These soft white cheeses like cottage cheese and quark contain 8.5 percent protein and 7.5 percent fats. They therefore fall into the crystal-producing category, especially the cream cheeses that have an even higher level of protein (15 percent). Yogurts produce crystals because of their many acids (lactic acid). If white sugar is added to these foods, this increases their acid production, hence the amount of crystalline wastes they produce.

Eggs

Eggs consist of 6.2 percent proteins. Although their quantity of fats is close to 5.5 percent, eggs, despite all that, are classified among the crystal-producing foods because proteins are the nutrient present in the largest quantities. In combination with this are the phosphoric and sulfuric acids of the yolks, which are acidic. Because of the cholesterol they contain, they are secondary producers of colloidal wastes.

Mushrooms

Mushrooms do not contain a high quantity of proteins, but practice has shown that they are producers of crystalline wastes. This comes from the proteins they do contain, purines, and acidic minerals such as phosphorus.

Food	Protein Content Percentage
Cultivated mushrooms	2.2%
Wild mushrooms	2.2%
Porcini	2.8%
Truffle	9%
Shitake	18%

Sugars and Sweets

Normally sugar does not produce any waste. It breaks down into energy and into water and carbon dioxide that are eliminated by the kidneys and lungs, respectively. Sugar is a clean energy only if it is properly metabolized. This is often not the case, especially when the sugar in question is white and refined. In fact, when it has been stripped of its vitamins and minerals by the refining process, it is not metabolized correctly. Its absorption into the tissues is interrupted at an acidic stage (lactic, pyruvic, succinic), therefore it forms crystals.

> Sugar is not a clean energy unless it can be properly metabolized.

Because of their high concentration of carbohydrates (99.5 percent) and the many acids that they can produce, refined white sugar and the food products that contain it are huge producers of crystalline wastes.

Food	Carbohydrate Content Percentage
Milk chocolate	55.6% (and 33.7% fat, which makes it a secondary producer of colloidal wastes)
Jelly (on average)	70.1%
Syrup	74%
Refined white sugar	99.5%

Honey (77 percent) and whole sugar (96 percent) retain all the vitamins, minerals, and trace elements that are provided by nature. Thus they will be metabolized properly. The same holds true for all fruits, including dried fruits (from 62 percent to 69 percent sugar). Despite their high sugar content, they produce very small amounts of waste because they are well metabolized.

Coffee, Tea, Cocoa
These drinks are rich in purines, the precursors for uric acid, a waste that is crystalline in nature.

Wine, Vinegar
Because of their rich acid content, wine and vinegar produce large amounts of crystals in the body.

COLLOIDAL AND CRYSTALLINE FOODS

Foods	Primarily	Secondarily
Cereals	Colloidal wastes	Crystals
Starchy foods	Colloidal wastes	
Cheeses	Colloidal wastes	Crystals
Milk	Colloidal wastes	
Oil, Fats	Colloidal wastes	
Oleaginous fruits	Colloidal wastes	Crystals
Beans	Colloidal wastes	Crystals
Animal meats	Crystals	Colloidal wastes
Eggs	Crystals	Colloidal wastes
Yogurt	Crystals	
Mushrooms	Crystals	
White sugar, sweets, jelly	Crystals	
Coffee, tea, cocoa, wine, vinegar	Crystals	

CONCLUSION

Depending on their composition, foods are suppliers of colloidal substances or crystals. More specifically, crystals are produced by proteins and acids while colloidal wastes are produced by carbohydrates and fats.

6

Drainage Methods

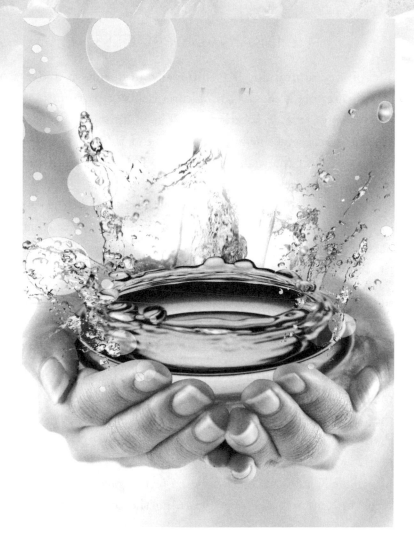

Because disease is due to the accumulation of toxins in the body's cellular terrain, the appropriate therapy is to drain these toxins out of the terrain.

THE DRAINAGE PROCESS

The process of draining is traditionally an operation undertaken to restore lands for agricultural fields or pastures that have become overly waterlogged. The draining is accomplished by the placement of underground tubes—drains—that will collect the water from the ground and facilitate its flow out of the field.

When applying this concept to the human body, the soil to be reclaimed is the physiological terrain; the waters that have accumulated there are the toxins that are overloading the body; and the drains are the eliminatory organs. These drains do not have to be installed as is the case in the field because the body already has them. These drains are the liver, the intestines, the kidneys, the skin, and the lungs. The main problem is that they are functioning too slowly and they are confronted by a quantity of toxins higher than those they can manage to eliminate, hence the clogging of the terrain. Thus they must be stimulated, which is to say their level of performance needs to be increased. This way they can start to function properly again (if their work was insufficient), and even above their normal pace, in order to catch up with the backlog. Draining the toxins from the body consists of stimulating the work level of the eliminatory organs, something that can be achieved in several different ways.

Draining the toxins from the body requires
stimulating the work level of the eliminatory organs.

The Specialized Eliminatory Organs

Given the fact that colloidal substances and crystals are different kinds of waste, they are not drained by the same organs. The eliminatory organs each have their specialty; some of them specialize in eliminating colloidal wastes, others eliminate crystals. When confronted by an outbreak of illness, it is not advisable to stimulate one eliminatory organ at random, or all of them at the same time. It is far more effective to choose those that correspond to the kinds of waste that are characterized by the illness.

For example, to treat acne, which is a colloidal disorder, the liver should be stimulated and not the kidneys, because the latter organ eliminates crystals, not colloidal wastes. The question of whether a disease is colloidal or crystalline has been discussed in chapter 4, and which eliminatory organs handle colloidal wastes or crystalline wastes was examined in chapter 3. Based on what kind of illness one is suffering from, it can be determined which eliminatory organ should be focused on in order to treat the disease.

There are several eliminatory organs that handle colloidal wastes, however, and several for crystals. In the case of arthritis, for example, a disease of crystal origin, how do we decide which is the best of the crystal-eliminating organs to encourage?

The Choice Between Principal and Secondary Eliminatory Organs

If a person is generally in good health, then in principle all the eliminatory organs corresponding to the wastes responsible for the disease could be stimulated together. There is a risk though that the body's forces will be scattered, causing an overall lowering of the body's ability to effectively eliminate wastes. This often proves to be the case, because individuals who need to treat an affliction are rarely at the top of their game, physiologically speaking, and are lacking strength and vitality. So it is much better to pick only one eliminatory organ to concentrate one's efforts on. It should obviously be the strongest organ that is selected. A hierarchy of these organs actually exists, based on their eliminatory capacities. A distinction is made between the principal eliminatory organs, which have very high capacities for filtering and eliminating wastes, and secondary eliminatory organs, which have lesser capabilities in this regard.

Of course the situation will be entirely different for someone who, although in good health, is aware of physiological weaknesses and wants to drain a precise kind of waste from the body as a preventive measure. This individual can stimulate several eliminatory organs without any risk or problem.

The recommendation to only stimulate one eliminatory organ at a time is limited to individuals who are run-down or have low vitality. As a rule, individuals in good health can stimulate several eliminatory organs simultaneously.

The hierarchy of the eliminatory organs is outlined in the table below.

Eliminatory Strength	Colloidal Wastes	Crystal Wastes
Principal	Liver, intestines	Kidneys
Secondary	Sebaceous glands, lungs	Sudoriferous glands

The liver and intestines earn their place as primary eliminatory organs for the removal of colloidal wastes for very specific reasons. The liver is the largest gland in the body. Its capacity for filtering and neutralizing colloidal wastes is enormous. The intestines, meanwhile, are the organs that evacuate the largest quantities of wastes (the stools). The quantity of colloidal substances expelled by the sebaceous glands is clearly much smaller, which ranks them in a secondary place. The same is true for the lungs, which specialize in the evacuation of gaseous wastes. They will only expel colloidal wastes out of necessity, when the other eliminatory organs are functioning poorly.

The kidneys sit at the top of the hierarchy of the eliminatory organs that expel crystalline wastes, because the quantity of wastes they eliminate is higher than that which the sudoriferous glands can expel.

✚ Expert Tips and Tricks

Choosing the principal eliminatory organ is easy when crystalline diseases are involved as there is only one: the kidneys. But how do we choose when the disease in question is of colloidal origin as the liver and the intestines both occupy the top place? There is no general answer for this question as everything depends on the individual. If a person has a tendency to be constipated, then the intestines are the organs that need to be stimulated first. If, on the other hand, the intestines are functioning properly, it is necessary to opt for stimulation of the liver. When in doubt, however, it is always a better idea to stimulate the liver. An abundant release of bile will have a laxative effect, and therefore a positive effect on the intestines. Stimulating the liver amounts to indirectly activating the intestines.

DIVERSION THERAPIES

The fact that there are several different eliminatory organs that specialize in removing each kind of waste—colloidal or crystalline—is a great help in treatment. This makes it possible to bring relief to an exhausted eliminatory organ by detouring the toxins to another organ of the same family. This procedure is called a diversion.

> Diverting is a way to provide relief to an exhausted eliminatory organ by directing the toxins to another organ of the same family.

The diversions are created by stimulating a particular eliminatory organ in a very intense fashion. The opening of a large exit portal from the body attracts the toxins to it. Some of the wastes that should have been eliminated by the sluggish organ are now drawn to the stimulated organ. The activation of this organ is achieved through taking hepatic or laxative plants and other herbs, depending on the individual case, and by techniques involving hydrotherapy, massage, and so forth.

Suppose someone is suffering from acute eczema caused by crystal waste. Should the elimination organ of the skin be stimulated, which will only make the inflammation worse? No, it is preferable to divert the toxins toward the kidneys, which also handle crystal wastes and are not suffering from any disorder. Another example would be taking herbs that promote expectoration during a case of bronchitis; often this only reinforces the problem because the lungs are already overworked by all the wastes with which they are overloaded. In a case like this, it is far preferable to divert the wastes somewhere else, toward the intestines or liver, by strongly stimulating these two organs. These two examples show how relief can be provided to a secondary eliminatory organ by diverting wastes to a primary organ. The opposite is also possible. Suppose one of the principal organs, the kidneys for example, is ailing greatly. Rather than compelling it to work harder, the skin can be stimulated by procedures that cause it to sweat abundantly (saunas, hot baths, and so forth). Of course in a situation like this the draining is not taking place through what is theoretically the strongest organ but through the one, given the circumstances, that is the most effective.

The means of stimulating the activity of the eliminatory organs and draining them of the toxins that have collected in the terrain are easy to apply. They will be presented here, one eliminatory organ after another, with sufficiently explicit instructions to enable the reader to independently put them to work. (Those wishing to learn more about detoxification should read my book *The Detox Mono Diet*.)

THE DRAINING OF THE COLLOIDAL ELIMINATORY ORGANS

The Liver

The intensification of the liver's ability to filter and eliminate wastes can be most easily brought about by the use of medicinal herbs, preferably organic, such as can be found in health stores and natural food markets. Their active properties increase the extraction of wastes from the bloodstream and encourage bile production and expulsion. They can be taken, according to personal preference, as infusions, mother tinctures, tablets, or gelcaps. The form in which they are taken is of little import as all these preparations are effective.

👆 **Good to Know**

The fundamental question is that of dosage. The general rule is to take as much as is needed, at three separate intervals during the day, to bring about an observable effect. In the case of hepatic herbs, its effect on the liver cannot be observed directly, but its effect can be seen, indirectly, in the intestines. The increased bile production caused by the hepatic herbs acts as a laxative because bile lubricates the intestines and stimulates intestinal peristalsis. This increase of intestinal eliminations (without it becoming too excessive) is the sign that the amount of herbs taken is sufficient. If the intestines exhibit no effect, the dosage should be increased. The dosages provided below are the average doses and can be adapted to individual needs.

Rosemary

Infusion: 1–2 teaspoons of rosemary leaves per cup, steeped for fifteen minutes, 3 cups a day

Mother tincture: 10–40 drops in water, three times a day

Tablets: Follow manufacturer's instructions—generally 1–2 tablets, with water, three times a day

Dandelion

Decoction: A large handful of leaves and roots per liter of water, boiled for two minutes then steeped for an additional ten minutes, 3 cups a day

Mother tincture: 10–50 drops in water, three times a day

Tablets: Follow manufacturer's instructions—generally
1–2 tablets, with water, three times a day

Boldo

Infusion: 1 teaspoon of the leaves per cup, steeped for ten
minutes, 3 cups a day
Mother tincture: 20–50 drops in water, three times a day
Tablets: Follow manufacturer's instructions—generally
1–3 tablets, with water, three times a day

Other Plants

- Artichoke
- Wild chicory
- Turmeric
- Centaury
- Black radish
- Goldenrod (solidago)
- Hepatic infusions or commercial liver-gallbladder teas

Hot Water Bottle

The hot water bottle is a rubber cushion that is filled with
hot water. By placing it over the liver—the right side of the
belly at the level of the bottom ribs—the hot water bottle
delivers a large amount of heat to the liver. The many blood
vessels crossing through this region begin to dilate, summon-
ing additional blood to the area. This results in the intensification of the filtration and elimination of colloidal wastes
by the liver. To be effective, the time the hot water bottle
should be left over the liver is about half an hour. It can be
repeated as many times as desired over the course of the day,

for example after meals, in the evening, or when getting ready to go to bed.

The Intestines

In order for the intestines, a major eliminatory organ that expels colloidal wastes, to function well, it is necessary for it to empty one or two times a day. This criterion alone is not enough though, the speed of intestinal transit is also quite important. This is normally from thirty-six to forty-eight hours. When the transit is too slow, the colloidal wastes it transports will either be reabsorbed by the body and collect in the cellular terrain or be directed to another eliminatory organ that handles this kind of waste.

> In order for the intestines, a major eliminatory organ that expels colloidal wastes, to function well, it is necessary for it to empty one or two times a day.

✚ Expert Tips and Tricks

The speed of the intestinal transit can be observed by eating foods that color the stools such as beets (red) and spinach (green).

The key to good intestinal elimination resides in the consumption of foods with high vegetable fiber. With their mass and their rough nature, fibers stimulate the peristaltic muscles whose rhythmic contractions are responsible for moving the bolus toward the end of the intestines.

In addition to the fiber supplied by diet, it can also be provided by taking:

- Wheat bran: 1–3 tablespoons a day, with water or in yogurt.
- Flaxseed: 1–2 tablespoons a day, with water or mixed in with food.
- Dried figs or prunes: Three to six pieces of fruit that have been soaked all day (or all night) in water. These should be eaten just before going to bed or upon getting up in the morning.

The following medicinal herbs are also highly effective.

Mallow

Infusion: 40 grams of leaves and/or flowers per liter of water, steeped for ten minutes, 3 cups a day
Mother tincture: 10–50 drops in water, three times a day
Tablets: Follow manufacturer's instructions—generally 1–2 tablets, with water, three times a day

Alder buckthorn (*Rhamnus frangula*)

Tea: It is rarely used this way because its flavor is so strong.
Mother tincture: 10–40 drops in water, three times a day.
Tablets: Follow manufacturer's instructions—generally 1–2 tablets, with water, three times a day.

Other Plants

- Cascara sagrada
- Cassia
- Hemp agrimony
- Licorice
- Polypody
- Commercial laxative or constipation teas

Enemas

The principle of enemas is the introduction of water into the intestines by way of the anus in order to soften the stools there. When an individual is constipated, it is because their stools are too dry. By virtue of the water supplied by the enema, these stools are liquefied and can be eliminated easily, as is the case with diarrhea.

Distinction is made between three kinds of enema, based on the amount of water used.

1. *The Rectal Douche:* This is the smallest enema. Only 3 deciliters (10 ounces) of water are injected into the anus with the aid of a bulb syringe that can be purchased at specialty shops. The purpose is not to introduce a large volume of water but to fill the rectal ampulla, the terminating end of the colon. The water is not held in but rejected immediately. By flowing out again, the water carries with it, by suction, the matter that is being held up higher in the intestines. The abrupt evacuation of water also triggers, as a reflexive action, intestinal peristalsis.

   A series of two or three rectal douches in a row

permits a good emptying of the intestines. The procedure is innocuous and can be practiced once a day over a two to three-week period.

2. *The 1–2 Liter Enema:* In this kind of enema, a greater quantity of water is used (1–2 liters). It fills the descending colon and part of the transverse colon. The water is intentionally retained for a period of five to ten minutes, so it can thoroughly liquefy the stools found there.

   To carry out this kind of enema, you will need to use a complete enema tub kit. This includes a receptacle for the water and a long rubber tube with a cannula at the end that has a faucet.

   The enema is applied in the following manner:

   - Fill the tub with water that is at body temperature and place it on an object slightly above you, a table for example.
   - Go on all fours and introduce the cannula into your anus with the faucet closed.
   - Lean your torso forward and open the faucet.
   - Breathe deeply to encourage the water to penetrate.
   - If the water pressure is too high or painful, stop the flow of liquid for one or two minutes by turning the faucet off.
   - Once all the water in the tub has entered your body, take out the cannula.
   - Keep the water in for five to ten minutes in order to give it enough time to soften the stools.
   - Sit on the toilet and let your intestines empty out.

A series of three enemas with an interval of two to three days between each one should allow for a thorough emptying and cleansing, accomplishing the elimination of many toxins.

3. *Colonic Irrigation:* During this procedure, several gallons of water will make a transit through the colon. To achieve this transit, the cannula contains two tubes. One is used to allow water to enter the body; the other lets it leave. A special device gently propels the water into the colon through one of the cannula's tubes; the other remains closed. The water intake continues this way until the colon is entirely filled. Once this has been achieved, the second tube of the cannula is opened to allow the water to leave. The first tube remains open to allow the intake of water to continue. This creates a water current entering and exiting the colon. As the water enters, an equivalent amount of waste-laden liquid comes out. This liquid transit has a scouring effect on the wastes that have collected and are often stuck to the walls of the colon. In this way the intestines are not only freed of recent wastes but also those that have accumulated over the long term because of poor intestinal elimination.

The necessity for a complex apparatus to perform colonic irrigations means that the cure can only be handled by a therapist experienced in the use of such a device. An excellent emptying of the colon can be obtained in one or two appointments.

Drink More

Following the same idea, the intake of fluids can be performed orally. By drinking more water than usual (2.5–3.5 liters a day), you can increase the quantity of liquid available for softening the stools in the intestines.

Whey

Whey (for more see my book *The Whey Prescription*) has gentle but effective laxative properties. Sold as a powder, it only needs to be mixed with water (1–2 tablespoons per glass of water) to reconstitute liquid whey. You should drink one to five glasses of this a day.

The Sebaceous Glands

The body releases sebum continuously over the course of the day. In order to intensify their working rhythm—and thereby their elimination of colloidal wastes—it is necessary to apply heat. This accelerates the blood circulation and lymphatic circulation in these glands. There are different means for obtaining this result.

- Intense physical exercise that produces heat and causes perspiration will push the sebaceous gland to produce more sebum.
- Hot baths, Turkish baths, and saunas have a visible effect of causing perspiration, but they also stimulate sebum secretion.

Certain medicinal herbs are recommended to support the work of the sebaceous glands.

Wild Pansy (*Viola tricolor*)

Tea: 60 grams of flowers per liter of water, steeped for ten minutes, 3 cups a day

Mother tincture: 50 drops in water, three times a day

Tablets: Follow manufacturer's instructions—generally 1–2 tablets, with water, three times a day

Burdock

Decoction: 40 grams of roots per liter of water, boiled ten minutes, 3 cups a day

Mother tincture: 30–40 drops in water, three times a day

Tablets: Follow manufacturer's instructions—generally 1–2 tablets, with water, three times a day

Other Plants

- Borage

The Lungs

The colloidal wastes that clog the bronchial tubes can be dislodged by the breathlessness caused by sustained physical effort. The intense in and out movement of the air, added to the repeated dilations and contractions of the bronchial tubes and alveoli facilitate the expulsion of mucous materials. This can be achieved by a brisk jog, a session of gymnastic exercises, a bike ride, and so forth.

Medicinal herbs that act on the respiratory tract are also of great assistance. They make the colloidal wastes and secretions more fluidic. By making these wastes less sticky, they ease their elimination from the body. Medicinal herbs also dilate the pulmonary alveoli, the little sacs at the extreme tips of the bronchial tree, in which colloidal wastes can easily be lodged. This increase in fluidity also takes place in the upper respiratory tract: the nose, throat, and sinus.

Thyme

Tea: 1 teaspoon of leaves and flowers per cup of water, steeped for ten minutes, 3 cups a day

Mother tincture: 20–40 drops in water, three times a day

Tablets: Follow manufacturer's instructions—generally 1–2 tablets, with water, three times a day

Eucalyptus

Tea: 3–4 leaves per cup of water, steeped for fifteen minutes, 3 cups a day

Mother tincture: 40–50 drops in water, three times a day

Tablets: Follow manufacturer's instructions—generally 1–2 tablets, with water, three times a day

Other Plants

- Oregano
- Plantain
- Scots pine
- Licorice
- Coltsfoot

The Dry Cure for the Elimination of Colloidal Wastes

As a general rule, the colloidal wastes that should be removed from the extracellular fluid are too voluminous to cross through the walls of the blood capillaries so they can enter the bloodstream and be transported to the eliminatory organs.

So how, then, are they eliminated? They are eliminated, not by the bloodstream but through the lymphatic system. The colloidal wastes enter the lymphatic vessels. These vessels carry them to the lymph nodes where they are reduced into smaller particles. The reduced size of these wastes now allows them to enter the bloodstream, which they do at the level of the subclavicle veins. From there these colloidal substances are transported to the liver or another eliminatory organ that handles these kinds of wastes.

The elimination of colloidal wastes by the lymphatic system is slow. The 5 to 6 liters of lymph contained in the network of the lymphatic vessels only spills into the blood at a rate of 1 liter every twenty-four hours. This is almost nothing in comparison to the blood, which travels through the body, and also through the eliminatory organs, in a matter of minutes.

Means do exist for accelerating the circulation of lymph, however. One of them is based on the fact that the body is constantly seeking to maintain blood volume at a very specific level. When this volume is reduced, the body triggers thirst so we will drink, causing the blood volume to return to normal. If the signal to drink is left unheeded, another process will be set in motion. The circulation of lymph will accelerate so that the water of which it is made will spill into the bloodstream in greater quantity to restore its standard volume. Depending on the extent of the dehydration, this acceleration can multiply the speed with which the lymph fluid is spilled into the bloodstream by two, three, or even four times. In this way it will no longer be the standard liter of lymph a day that spills into the bloodstream, but 3 or 4 liters, with all the wastes they contain.

It is this physiological process that is used to best advantage in the dry cure. This cure consists of intentionally avoiding the ingestion of any liquid for a certain period of time. The blood will inevitably shrink in volume, because the daily eliminations of water by urine and sweat are no longer being replaced by fresh supplies. When the blood volume shrinks, the body's defense system, which consists of accelerating the flow of lymph, will be set in motion.

⚠ Caution!

It would be a mistake to think that the longer this treatment is imposed the more effective it will be. The body cannot tolerate a prolonged period of dehydration. To go several days, from three to less than six, without drinking poses a serious threat and eventually leads to death. A dry cure is a therapeutic action only and not a healthy lifestyle. It is therefore critical that it be restricted to last for only a short time.

In concrete terms, it consists of ingesting no fluids for twenty-four hours. This means not only avoiding beverages but also foods with high water content. It so happens that most foods consist of large amounts of liquid.

Food	Water Content
Fruits	80%–90%
Vegetables	80%–96%
Meat	60%–70%
Dairy products	30%–80%

The available selection of truly dry foods, on the other hand, is quite limited.

Food	Water Content
Grains	12%
Toast	7%–8%
Oleaginous fruits	3%–5%
Cookies, crackers	3%
Corn flakes	3%

Consuming only foods like this will soon cause you to become thirsty so a complete fast is often easier to follow.

✪ Expert Tips and Tricks

Before undertaking a dry cure, you should go through a wet cure during which you drink a large amount. The role of this wet cure is to purify the blood and thoroughly cleanse the eliminatory organs in order to prepare them to receive the toxins that the dry cure will force to rise out of the depths of the body.

The day before taking the cure it is good to take a laxative to empty the intestines. It is also necessary to drink less than you normally would. Conversely, the day after the dry cure, you should drink copiously: 3 to 4 liters of water. The wastes that the lymph has released into the bloodstream have now collected in the eliminatory organs. The huge intake of liquid will apply pressure to the filters of these organs and facilitate the expulsion of these wastes. To have any real results you should wait two weeks and then repeat the cure. Do this one or two more times as needed.

Other Means for Draining Lymph

In addition to the dry cure, other methods exist for stimulating the drainage of lymph to remove colloidal wastes, both on a regular basis and when additional cleansing is desired.

Physical Exercise

The contractions of the muscle caused by physical effort as well as the intensification of respiratory movement greatly increase the speed of blood circulation. The strong current of blood that this moves into the subclavian veins—the site connected to the lymph system and which receives the released lymph—results in the increased suction of lymph into this blood flow. The lymph will spill more quickly onto the bloodstream, along with the colloidal wastes it carries. Regular physical exercise for prolonged periods is therefore a powerful means of ridding the body of its colloidal wastes.

> Regular physical exercise for prolonged periods is a powerful means of ridding the body of its colloidal wastes.

Lymphatic Drainage

Perfected by Emil Vodder (1896–1986), this extremely gentle massage, which works by applying light, circular pressure on the course of the lymph vessels and lymph nodes, can accelerate the release of lymph by three times. It is best to seek out the assistance of someone who has been trained in this method to get optimal results.

THE DRAINAGE OF THE ELIMINATORY ORGANS THAT HANDLE CRYSTALLINE WASTES

The Kidneys

Taking medicinal herbs with diuretic properties will increase both the volume of urine the body eliminates and its concentration of toxins. The quantity of uric acid, urea, and so on extracted from the blood by the renal filter is therefore higher than normal, thanks to the active properties of these plants.

Heather

> *Decoction–Tea:* 1 tablespoon of flowering tops per liter of water, boiled for three minutes then steeped for ten minutes, 3 cups a day
>
> *Mother tincture:* 20–50 drops in water, three times a day
>
> *Tablets:* Follow manufacturer's instructions—generally 1–2 tablets, with water, three times a day

Bearberry

> *Tea:* A handful of leaves and flowers per liter of water, steeped for fifteen minutes, 3 cups a day

Mother tincture: 20–40 drops in water, three times a day

Tablets: Follow manufacturer's instructions—generally 1–2 tablets, with water, three times a day

Other plants

- Linden (sapwood)
- Birch
- Blackcurrant (leaves)
- Cherry (stems)
- Couch grass
- Ash
- Onion
- Nettle
- Mouse-ear hawkweed (*Hieracium pilosella*)
- Horsetail
- Commercial diuretics or kidney-bladder teas

Whey

In addition to its laxative properties, which we noted earlier, whey has a strong diuretic effect. This can be achieved by drinking five glasses of reconstituted whey at different intervals over the course of the day (1–2 tablespoons of whey powder per glass of water).

Water

Water is more than just a support fluid for the elimination of wastes. When it is low in minerals, it has the ability to catch the crystal wastes in the terrain. It therefore becomes laden with more substantial amounts of crystals than water that already has a number of suspended substances in it, such as mineral water and tap water. This property can be used to advantage when draining crystal wastes from the body. If a person following the drainage cure chooses the low-mineral bottled waters that are commercially available, when drinking the 2.5 liters of water per day the amount of crystals that are drained will be increased.

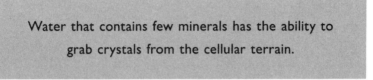

Water that contains few minerals has the ability to grab crystals from the cellular terrain.

Filtered water can also be used for this purpose. In fact, the use of commercial filters to purify water has the side effect of making this water's mineral content substantially lower. This water will capture more crystal wastes from the body's cellular terrain. The degree of purification depends on the filter.

Water is considered to have low mineral content if it contains less than 50 milligrams of minerals per liter. This is the case for the following waters.

WATERS WITH LOW MINERAL CONTENT

Name of Water	mg/liter
United States	
Hawaii Water	0.005 mg
Rain	1.5 mg
Thunder Mountain	8 mg

Name of Water	mg/liter
Famous Premium Drinking Water	9 mg
Sparkletts	18 mg
Ice Mountain	19 mg
Snow Line	19 mg
Ozarder	23 mg
Great Bear	24 mg
Snow Valley	29 mg
Arbutus	31–61 mg
Ozarka	32 mg
Canada	
Ice Age	4 mg
Arctic Glacier	10 mg
Spirit Water	10 mg
Sugarloaf Spring Rain	23 mg
Sun Spring eau de Glacier	40 mg
Whistler Water Pure Glacial Spring	48 mg
France	
Mont Roucous	18.1 mg
Montcalm	20 mg
Mont-Doré	27 mg
Montagne d'Arée	36 mg
Charrier	37 mg
Fontaine de la Reine	40 mg
Isabelle	42 mg
Celtic	46 mg

Name of Water	mg/liter
Belgium	
Spa Reine	33 mg
Spa Barisat	49 mg
Switzerland	
San Clemente	44 mg
Italy	
Lavretana	13.9 mg
Amorosa	20.2 mg
Fonte della Al	21.2 mg
Monviso	30 mg
Fonte Santa Barbara	35.4 mg
San Bernardo Sorgente Rocciaviva	38 mg
Bernina	39.2 mg
Daggio	44.5 mg
Valmora	48 mg
Spain	
Agua de Quess	26.8 mg
Bezoya	27 mg
Portugal	
Glaciar	16 mg
Aurora	19 mg
Fontes	20 mg
Setefontes	20 mg
Alardo	25.4 mg
Agua de Marao	27 mg

Name of Water	mg/liter
Serra da Estrela	27 mg
Nascente Salutis	30.4 mg
Agua do Fastio	33.7 +\- 4 mg
Serrana	44 mg
Australia	
Rain Farm	1 mg
Lithgow Valley	16 mg
Linton Park	35 mg
Crystal Organic Water	49 mg

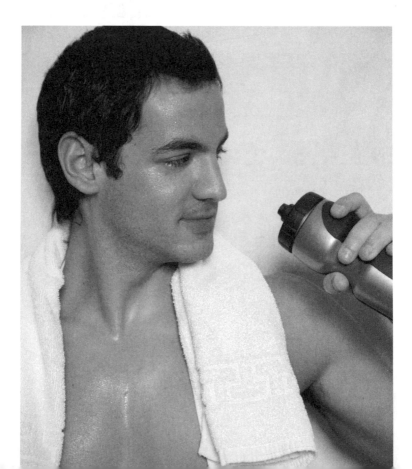

Skin

Causing the skin to perspire is the most effective method for draining crystalline wastes through it. An intensification of the labor performed by the sudoriferous glands can be obtained by:

- Intensive physical effort
- All sports activities
- Taking hot baths
- Sauna
- Turkish bath

✛ Expert Tips and Tricks

It is a good idea to drink a lot before doing one of these activities to provide a strong support for the transport and elimination of crystalline wastes. The use of medicinal herbs with sweat-inducing properties makes it possible to intensify the work performed by the sudoriferous glands.

Elder flowers

Tea: 1 tablespoon of flowers per cup of water, steeped for ten minutes, 3 cups a day

Linden

Tea: 30 grams of leaves per liter of water, steeped for ten minutes, 3 cups a day

Chamomile

Tea: 5–10 flowers per cup of water, steeped for ten minutes, 3 cups a day

Other Plants

- Burdock
- Borage
- Wild pansy

One Additional Procedure for Draining Crystals

Along with the prior methods discussed for stimulating and draining toxins from the kidneys and the skin, a process for the neutralization of acids that have collected in the tissues of the body is quite useful.

Alkaline Food Supplements

Acids as a general rule form part of the family of crystalline wastes. These crystals collected in the terrain can only rise quite slowly back into the bloodstream, where they can next be carried to the appropriate eliminatory organs. The reason for this is that a large influx of acid into the blood will alter its pH (its degree of acidity), which is harmful to the health and the survival of the organism.

Consequently, the acids can only be released from the tissues once they have been neutralized by an alkaline substance. The combination of an acid and an alkaline creates a neutral salt. Because of its neutrality, this salt does not alter the blood pH. To make it possible for more acids than normal to rise back into the bloodstream from the depths of the cellular terrain, it is therefore necessary to provide the body with alkaline substances. This means adding alkaline minerals as a supplement to those that are normally provided by diet. The acids neutralized by these alkaline minerals can then harmlessly enter the bloodstream in the form of neutral salts to be eliminated from the body.

There are alkaline mineral preparations available. These are dietary alkaline supplements that can be found commercially. The minerals of these alkaline blends are easy for the body to incorporate. For dosage, check the manufacturer's instructions. (To get more information on this important topic, see my book *The Acid-Alkaline Diet for Optimum Health*.)

CONCLUSION

The eliminatory organs specialize in the removal of either colloidal wastes or crystalline wastes. The eliminatory organs that handle colloidal substances are the liver, intestines, sebaceous glands, and the lungs; those dealing with crystals are the kidneys and the sudoriferous glands.

7

Regulating Your Food Intake

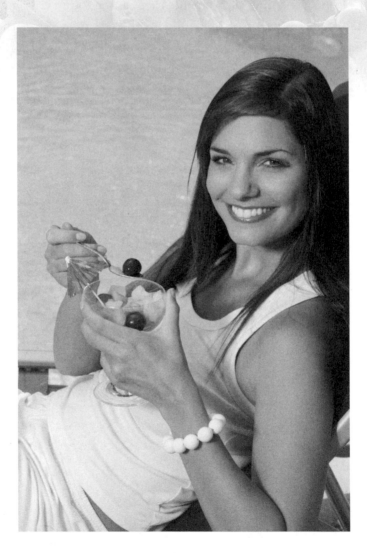

Once it has been determined whether the illness in question is of colloidal or crystalline origin, it is necessary to correct the diet. The food intake should be reduced to spare the body having to deal with the constant arrival of new colloidal or crystalline substances. This amounts to eliminating the cause of the illness, which will cause its symptoms to vanish of their own accord.

To apply these dietary corrections, it is essential to first review your standard menu.

THE STANDARD MENU

A standard menu is simply a menu that is truly representative of what an individual normally eats. Of course, most people eat different things every day; or so it may seem. In reality though, despite their varied appearances, the meals tend to resemble each other and can be broken down to two or three basic variations.

To establish a standard menu, it is necessary to document one's dietary habits. You should note everything that is consumed during the course of the day: on getting up, at breakfast, midmorning snack, lunch, afternoon tea, dinner, and before going to bed. Furthermore, some people snack quite a bit between meals. This must also be accounted for as it can represent a large amount of different foods.

✚ Expert Tips and Tricks

To maintain a clear view of the menu, it is a good idea not to get overly bogged down in the details. Initially in any case there is no need to specify if the meats consumed are beef or pork, simply summarize it as *meat*. You could also use the terms *cooked* or *raw* vegetables without explicitly stating what vegetable was eaten.

Here is an example of a standard menu. The variants of a specific meal are separated by the word *or*.

EXAMPLE: STANDARD MENU

6:30 a.m.		black coffee, no sugar
7:00 a.m.		whole grain bread + butter + jam + one orange juice + two coffees with milk and one sugar
	or	cereal + milk + two teas with milk and two sugars
9:00 a.m.		black tea with milk and two sugars + three or four cookies
	or	black tea with milk and two sugars + one croissant
12:00 noon		raw and cooked vegetables + pasta (or rice) + meat + fruit salad + one cup of coffee + water
	or	salami sandwich + soda
4:00 p.m.		chocolate + one tea with sugar
	or	pastry + one tea with sugar
7:00 p.m		fish + cooked vegetables + potatoes + water
	or	dark bread + cheese + cold cuts + two glasses beer (or wine)

or	vegetable soup + cheese + dark bread + water
10:00 p.m.	chocolate + water

ANALYSIS OF THE STANDARD MENU

Once the standard menu has been established, it should next be analyzed. Depending upon the colloidal or crystalline nature of the illness to be treated, the emphasis will be placed on the foods that produce either colloidal wastes or crystals and whether they are primary or secondary sources of these wastes. They are producing the wastes in question in either case.

The two tables that follow illustrate how to proceed. Both tables use the standard menu provided above but in the first the foods with colloidal wastes are underlined and in the second the foods producing crystals are emphasized.

COLLOIDAL FOODS ON THE STANDARD MENU

6:30 a.m.	black coffee, no sugar
7 a.m.	whole grain bread + butter + jam + one orange juice + two coffees with milk and one sugar
or	cereal + milk + two teas with milk and two sugars
9:00 a.m.	black tea with milk and two sugars + three or four cookies
or	black tea with milk and two sugars + one croissant
12:00 p.m.	raw and cooked vegetables + pasta (or rice) + meat + fruit salad + one cup of coffee + water
or	salami sandwich + soda

COLLOIDAL FOODS ON THE STANDARD MENU
(continued)

4:00 p.m.	<u>chocolate</u> + one tea with sugar
or	<u>pastry</u> + one tea with sugar
7:00 p.m.	fish + cooked vegetables + <u>potatoes</u> + water
or	<u>dark bread</u> + <u>cheese</u> + <u>cold cuts</u> + two glasses wine
or	vegetable soup + <u>cheese</u> + <u>dark bread</u> + water
10:00 p.m.	<u>chocolate</u> + water

CRYSTAL FOODS ON THE STANDARD MENU

6:30 a.m.	<u>black coffee</u>, no sugar
7:00 a.m.	<u>whole grain bread</u> + butter + <u>jam</u> + one <u>orange</u> juice + two <u>coffees</u> with milk and one <u>sugar</u>
or	<u>cereal</u> + milk + two <u>teas</u> with milk and two <u>sugars</u>
9:00 a.m.	<u>black tea</u> with milk and two <u>sugars</u> + three or four <u>cookies</u>
or	<u>black tea</u> with milk and two <u>sugars</u> + one <u>croissant</u>
12:00 a.m.	raw and cooked vegetables + <u>pasta</u> (or <u>rice</u>) + <u>meat</u> + fruit salad + one cup of <u>coffee</u>, no sugar + water
or	<u>salami sandwich</u> + <u>soda</u>
4:00 p.m.	<u>chocolate</u> + one <u>tea</u> with <u>sugar</u>
or	<u>pastry</u> + one <u>tea</u> with <u>sugar</u>
7:00 p.m.	<u>fish</u> + cooked vegetables + potatoes + water
or	<u>dark bread</u> + <u>cheese</u> + <u>cold cuts</u> + two glasses wine
or	vegetable soup + <u>cheese</u> + <u>dark bread</u> + water
10:00 p.m.	<u>chocolate</u> + water

The analysis starts by asking the following questions.

1. **Is there one food that is consumed in quantities significantly higher than the other foods?** If so, this is the culprit responsible for the supply of colloidal or crystalline wastes. It is enough to sharply reduce the consumption of this food item to see a reduction in the production of the colloidal or crystal wastes responsible for the disease. For example, some people eat a noticeably large portion of meat, pasta, chocolate, cake, or pastry at mealtimes.

2. **Is there a food that is eaten in normal amounts but eaten numerous times during the day?** It would appear that food eaten in small quantities produces little waste. However, the repeated ingestion of this food item over the course of the day adds up so in the final analysis it constitutes a large quantity. This could be bread, for example, which not only forms a basic part of breakfast every day (toast with butter and jelly) and a croissant or bagel for midmorning snack but also often accompanies the noon and evening meals.

   As another example, white sugar may appear at 7:00 a.m. in the jam, at 9:00 a.m. in a chocolate bar, at noon in dessert, in the cookies eaten at 4:00 p.m., and in the caramel custard that follows dinner as dessert, not to mention the sugar that is added to the coffee and tea drunk over the course of the day.

3. **Is there a kind of food (grains, meats) that is eaten frequently over the course of the day?** This question differs from the previous question in that it concerns

a type of food and not only one particular food. For example, dairy products can appear at every meal, but in different forms such as:

At 7:00 a.m. a yogurt; 9:00 a.m. a small cheese sandwich; 12:00 p.m. cottage cheese; 4:00 p.m. vanilla cream pudding; and at 7:00 p.m. aged cheeses eaten with bread.

As another example, some people eat ham at breakfast, meat at noon, and fish at night, thus consuming meats that are great producers of crystals three times a day.

By trying to answer these three questions you can discover the food or foods that are the primary culprits responsible for the health problem. The next step is changing the diet to correct this.

REGULATING THE DIET

The food or foods responsible should be restricted, because a reduction of their intake will bring about a reduction of the quantity of wastes they contribute to the body. This restriction can be more or less strict depending on the individual case.

Bringing It Back to Normal

This means that the foods that are being eaten in too large quantity are brought down to normal consumption levels. For example, rather than eating two fried eggs at breakfast every day, the individual might have a single egg, as is more common. A 7-ounce serving of meat would be reduced to

5 ounces, 10 ounces of pasta would be reduced to 7 ounces, and so forth. When it is the frequency with which the food is eaten that is the problem (see the example of bread, above), the food item in question will no longer be eaten at every meal but at a single meal, for example breakfast.

Reducing It Below Normal

The restriction here is stricter than in the preceding example because the food intake no longer meets normal needs but is below them. This also means that the production of wastes will be lower than before, which will enable the body to catch up with the backlog more easily. By not having to eliminate as many daily wastes, the body can work more on clearing out the ones that have collected in the terrain.

In practice, the individual will eat an intentionally set amount of the food item, for example half the normal portion: 1 tablespoon of butter instead of 2 per day, one slice of bread rather than two or three, and so on.

The Complete Elimination of the Food Item from the Diet

Some foods can be eliminated entirely. Because they are no longer being consumed, the wastes they produce will no longer be supplied to the body. This means the terrain will be more rapidly cleansed of that kind of waste, because the body's efforts to eliminate these toxins will no longer be hampered by incoming wastes.

⚠ Caution!

Complete elimination of a basic food item from the diet is always restricted to a set period of time as the body cannot be forever deprived of a food it needs in order to function properly. While temporary abstaining is possible, for perhaps several days to several weeks, a longer-lasting abstinence will inevitably cause deficiencies. This will mean that the existing problems caused by excess toxins will be complicated by deficiencies of vitamins, minerals, or other vital substances.

A dieting period should always be followed by a reintroduction of the food in question. This food must not be eaten in too high a quantity, though, but in a quantity adapted to the individual's metabolic capacities. The right quantity can be determined through trial and error: if it is too high, there will be an excess production of wastes causing the reappearance of the symptoms.

Certain foods that can be eliminated once and for all from the diet are the fake foods, meaning the foods created by man. These would include white sugar, highly refined flour, chocolate, candies, and so forth.

Certain foods that can be eliminated once and for all from the diets are the fake foods, meaning the foods created by man—white sugar, highly refined flour, chocolate, candies, and so forth.

While it is normal, at the beginning, for the regulation of the diet to be fairly restrictive, it should subsequently, once the terrain has been cleansed of the bulk of the toxins, be modified to deal with the new circumstances. Going forward, its purpose is to ensure that the food intake is optimally balanced with the body's needs and its eliminatory capacities.

In this way toxins will no longer accumulate, and, because of that, the terrain will no longer deteriorate. The terrain will be healthy and offer the person who takes care of it plenty of vitality and good health.

CONCLUSION

Because colloidal and crystalline wastes are of food origin, it is essential to reduce the intake of the foods that are producing the wastes—colloidal or crystalline—that are responsible for the illness.

Conclusion

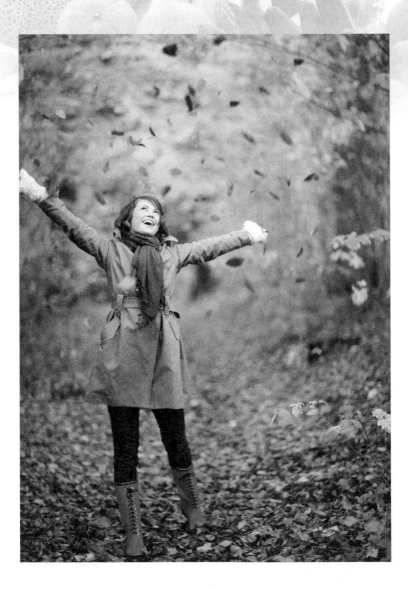

Health is not the work of fate, so it should not be left to chance. This has been clearly expressed by Doctor Paul Carton (1875–1947), one of the great pioneers of natural medicine.

> Human life does not unfold by the blind whim of exterior circumstances. A set of general and particular laws guides each of our lives. Knowing these laws exactly and applying them as precisely as possible, is the sole secret to happiness and health.

Among these is the law of cause and effect, meaning that everything (for example an accumulation of toxins in the physiological terrain) automatically brings about an effect (illness). Applying this law, it logically follows that the elimination of the illness (effects) can be obtained only by eliminating the cause (the toxins that created it). This is exactly what the cures offered in this book do. These treatments have a dual effect on the causes inasmuch as they reduce both the toxins that are burdening the terrain and the source of the toxins (an unsuitable dietary intake).

The beneficial results of these cures are explained by their conformity with natural law. Instead of contesting this law, they are sustained and reinforced by it. Knowing and applying these laws as precisely as possible is fundamental. This is where the true key to health can be found.

Index

Page numbers in *italics* refer to illustrations.

acetoacetic acid, 31

acne, 78–79, 84, 125

alder buckthorn, 134

alkaline food supplements, 152–53

allergies, 104

anxiety, 43, 44

arteriosclerosis, 12, 82

arthritis, 88–94, *89*

asthma, 76–77, 106

bacteria, 47

beans, 114–15

bearberry, 145–46

beta-hydroxybutyric acid, 31

bile and bile stones, 39–44, 103

blood, 6–7, *8*, 58–59

blood circulation, 44, 80–81

blood pressure, 60, 65, 82–83

blood thinners, 29

body fluids, 6–8, *8*, 11

boils, 79

boldo, 132

bones, 92

bronchial tree, 54–55

bronchitis, 11, 75, 106

burdock, 139

canaliculi, 40

canker sores, 97

capillaries, 7

carbohydrates, 13, 28–29, 31, 48–49, 108–9, 114–15

carcinogens, 13

cardiovascular disease, 100

Carton, Paul, 20, 165

cells, 5–6, 9

cellulitis, 83–84

chamomile, 152

chapped skin, 86–87

cheese, 111–12, 119

chlorine, 32
cholesterol, 27–28
cilia, 55
circulatory system, 80–84
cocoa, 121
coffee, 15, 121
colds, 11, 72–74
colitis, 98–99
colloidal toxins, 2–3, 21–23
  characteristics of, 26–29,
    32–33
  dry cure for, 140–44
  eliminatory organs for, 38–56,
    41, 46, 52, 54
  food producers of, 109–15
  illnesses caused by, 72–84,
    99–106
  insolubility of, 35–38
  membranes and, 25–26
colonic irrigation, 49–50
congested liver, 40–41
constipation, 47, 102–3
creatinine, 31
crystalline toxins, 2–3, 21–23
  characteristics of, 29–33
  eliminatory organs for,
    57–66
  food producers of, 115–22
  illnesses caused by, 84–96,
    99–106
  membranes and, 25–26
  solubility of, 35–38
cysts, 79

dairy products, 119
dandelion, 131–32
degenerative diseases, 100–102
dehydration, 141
dental cavities, 97
Detox Mono Diet, The, 130
diarrhea, 11, 12, 47
diet, 13–15, 160–63. *See also*
  food
digestion, 13–14, 48–49, 96–97
discharge, 69–70
disease
  terrain and, 5–10
  toxins and, 11–13, 68–70
diversion therapies, 128–30
drainage
  of colloidal eliminatory organs,
    130–45
  of crystalline wastes, 145–53
  diversion therapies, 128–30
  process of, 124–28
dry asthma, 106
dry bronchitis, 106
dry cough, 105

eczema, 11, 12, 78, 86, 129
eggs, 119
elder flowers, 151
elimination, insufficient, 14
eliminatory organs, 3, 15–16
  for colloidal wastes, 38–56, *41,*
    46, 52, 54
  for crystalline toxins, 57–66

drainage and, 125–28
mixing of toxins in, 104–5
solubility and, 35–38
See also drainage
enemas, 135–37
eucalyptus, 140
exercise, 19, 144
extracellular serum, 6–7, *8*

fats, 12, 13, 108–9, 112–13
colloidal substances from,
27–28
crystalline toxins from, 31
in stools, 48–49
fiber, 48, 133–34
figs, 134
fish, 117
flaxseed, 134
flocculates, 28
food, 3
colloidal toxins from, 109–15
crystalline toxins from,
115–22
overview of, 108–9
regulating, 160–63
standard menu, 155–60
food additives, 14, 39

gallbladder, 40–41, 43, 103
gallbladder flushes, 11
gastritis, 97
gout, 30, 94–95
grains, 109–11

hay fever, 104
health, terrain and, 9–10
heart attacks, 12, 83
heather, 145
heavy metals, 39
hemogliasis, 80–81
hemorrhoids, 11, 81–82
herbs, 130–33, 134, 145–46,
151–52
herpes, 87
high blood pressure, 82–83,
100
Hippocrates, 20
hives, 85–86
hot water bottles, 132–33
hydration, 65–66
hydrotherapy, 19

insecticides, 14
insolubility, 35–38
intestinal fermentation, 14
intestinal filter, 50–51
intestines, 15–16, 36, 44–48, *46*,
125, 137–39
intracellular fluid, 6–7, *8*
itching, 85

joints, 12, 87–95

kidneys, 14, 16, 36, 57–62, *57*,
95, 125–26, 145–47
kidney stones, 62, 95
Kousmine, Catherine, 21

lactic acid, 31, 96
lesions, 30
linden, 151
liver, 14, 15, 36, 38–44, *41*, 97–98, 125, 130–33
lungs, 16, 53–56, *54*, 125, 139–40
lymph and lymphatic system, 6–8, *8*, 144–45

mallow, 134
Marchesseau, Pierre-Valentin, 22
massage, 19
meat, 115–18
medications, 39
medicinal plants, 19, 131, 139–40, 145–46
membranes, 25–26, 50–51
minerals, 31–32
mucus, 26–27
muscles, 95
mushrooms, 120

Naturopathic Way, The, 16
nephrons, 58–59, *59*, 62–63
nerves, 95
neuritis, 95–96
nutrient utilization, 14
nuts, 113–14

Oddi sphincter, 44
oils, 112–13
organelles, 6

osteoarthritis, 93–94
overeating, 13, 14, 44, 51
overload, 10, 18–19
oxalic acid, 31

pain, 70–72
perspiration, 36, 64–65
pesticides, 39
phlegm, 12, 26, 55
phosphorus, 32
pimples, 11, 12
pollution, 15
proteins, 13, 31, 48–49, 108–9, 110, 114, 115–18
prunes, 134
pyruvic acid, 31

respiratory tract, 36, *54*, 72–77
ringworm, 103–4
rosemary, 131

salt, 13
sand, 62
saunas, 130
seafood, 117
sebaceous glands, 36, 51–53, *52*, 77–80, 125, 138–39
sedentary lifestyle, 43, 44
seeds, 113–14
Seignalet, Jean, 21
shingles, 87
sinusitis, 11, 74–75
skin, 16, 77–80, 84–87, 151–52

solubility, 35–38
spit, 26
standard menu, 155–60
starches, 28–29
stimulants, 15
stones, 62
stools, 26–27, 48–50
stress, 43, 44, 65
strokes, 12, 83
sudoriferous glands, 36, 62–66, 63, 125
sugar, 13, 120–21
sulfur, 32
sweating, 20, 64–65
sweets, 120–21
Sydenham, Thomas, 20

tea, 15, 121
tendonitis, 96
terrain
    chronic disease and, 102
    eliminating overload, 18–19
    explanation of, 5–9
    factors affecting, 14–15
    health and, 9–10
thyme, 140
tobacco, 15
tongue, white coating on, 46
toxins, 2–3
    characteristics of, 32–33
    disease and, 11–13
    eliminating overload, 18–19

eliminatory organs and, 38–66
    healing and, 19–21
    origins of, 13–15
    shutting off source, 17–18
    therapy for, 16–19
    types of, 21–23
    See also colloidal toxins; crystalline toxins
triglycerides, 28

urea, 10, 31
uric acid, 10, 13, 16, 31, 62
urinary issues, 12–13
urine, 57, 60, 61–62

vaginal mucous membranes, 36
varicose veins, 81
vinegar, 121
vitamins, 9
Vodder, Emil, 145
vomiting, 12

wastes, elimination of, 15–16
water, 47, 61, 138, 146–50
wheat bran, 134
whey, 138, 146
wild pansy, 139
wine, 121

yeast, 103–4
yogurt, 119